Putting Feminism to Work

"Suzanne Egan's work brings the insights of practice and theory together to understand how sexual assault services think about and use feminist knowledges. This book is a careful and creative exploration of spaces beyond slogans and polarities such as 'feminist or not' and 'medicalisation as oppressive.' In illuminating the intertwined and complex lived relationships between 'bodies, emotions, and institutions' to enhance our responses to those who have experienced sexual assault, Egan does indeed put feminism to work with rigour and passion."

—JaneMaree Maher, Professor, *Centre for Women's Studies & Gender Research, Sociology, Monash University*

"This book, aptly titled, successfully counters the assertions that feminism has lost its way and declined in influence. Egan illustrates how frontline workers, service providers, academics and policy makers working in sexual assault, have utilised and built on feminist knowledges so successfully that this knowledge is now taken for granted and routinely adopted. This is a beautifully written, inspiring book that, interweaving biography, history and meticulous research, generated many 'a ha' moments."

—Jane Mears, Associate Professor, *School of Social Sciences, Western Sydney University*

"This is an immensely important book for those of us who are feminists working within the apparatus of the state. Drawing on original research data and conceptualising feminism as a form of knowledge, Egan offers a masterful scholarly challenge to conventional feminist arguments that change is possible only through subversive political action outside the state. Arguing for the robustness and adaptability of feminism, she shows how feminism has become central and authoritative in our sexual assault services and sexual assault counsellors actively and productively put 'trauma' to work as part of contemporary feminist practice. Breathing new life into the old feminist catch-cry that the 'personal is political', Egan recognises the complexity of feminist knowledge, practices and interventions challenging the status quo and supporting individuals with the embodied effects of sexual violence. In doing so, this book makes a significant contribution to feminist knowledge by legitimising institutionalised feminism as an important component of feminist efforts, political activism and commitment to gender equality and structural social change."

—Mayet Costello, *Policy Manager in Violence, Abuse and Neglect Integration and Former Sexual Assault Counsellor*

Suzanne Egan

Putting Feminism to Work

Theorising Sexual Violence, Trauma and Subjectivity

palgrave
macmillan

Suzanne Egan
University of Sydney
New South Wales, NSW, Australia

ISBN 978-3-030-22108-9 ISBN 978-3-030-22109-6 (eBook)
https://doi.org/10.1007/978-3-030-22109-6

This Palgrave Macmillan imprint is published by the registered company Springer Nature Switzerland AG.
The registered company address is: Gewerbestrasse 11, 6330 Cham, Switzerland

Acknowledgements

I want to acknowledge the debt owed to friends, family and colleagues for their support during the process of producing this book and to the benefactors of the Thomas and Ethel Mary Ewing Postdoctoral Fellowship which enabled me to have a period of uninterrupted to time to focus on this work, during my time at the University of Sydney. A heartfelt thank you to the sexual assault services and practitioners who participated in my research, for taking the time to share their knowledge, expertise and reflections on the field of sexual assault service provision. Finally, a thank you to Palgrave editor Nina Guttapalle and her predecessor Amelia Derkatsch for their patience and guidance through the publication process.

In this book I draw on some work that has been previously published and am grateful for permission to reproduce extracts from this work here: SAGE Publications for extracts from S. Egan (2016) sexual assault as trauma: A Foucauldian examination of knowledge practices in the field of sexual assault service provision *Feminist Review* 112, 95–112; Elsevier Publishing for extracts from S. Egan (2019) Excavating feminist knowledges and practices in the field of sexual assault service provision: An Australian case study. *Women's Studies International Forum*, 74(May–June), 169–178.

Contents

Abbreviations

AHRC	Australian Human Rights Commission
BPD	borderline personality disorder
CASAC	Child and Adolescent Sexual Abuse Counsellors
c-PTSD	complex post-traumatic stress disorder
CPU	Child Protection Unit
DSM	Diagnostic and Statistical Manual of Mental Health
ECAV	Education Centre Against Violence
FACS	Family and Community Services
FMS	false memory syndrome
ISN	Incest Services Network
NGO	non-governmental organisation
NSW	New South Wales
NSWRCC	NSW Rape Crisis Centre
PTSD	post-traumatic stress disorder
R&DVSA	Rape and Domestic Violence Services Australia
SRCC	Sydney Rape Crisis Collective
STI	sexually transmitted infections
WAIC	Women Against Incest Collective

CHAPTER 1

Introduction

Impetus

The late 1990s marked my entry into the world of women's health and sexual assault services. Freshly minted from a university degree, I could not believe my good luck when I got a position as a sexual assault worker with a local service in my hometown. I loved the feminist and gender studies subjects I had studied at university and looked on my new position as an extension of those studies, an opportunity to do feminist work 'at the coalface' so to speak. It was a workplace and an area of work in which I felt 'at home'. As an interview participant commented when I returned to this field of work some years later, this time as a researcher, it was a place where it was 'easy to be a feminist'. Despite (or perhaps because of) this, one of my clearest early memories of this period was asking at one of the weekly team meetings if we could discuss what it actually was that made our service a feminist service. The question had been puzzling me for some time. It was not that I doubted it *was* a feminist service or that we *were* indeed feminist workers. I guess I meant it was not a criticism masquerading as a question—'I don't think this service *really* is feminist'—but rather something about which I was genuinely curious. I could not quite put my finger on exactly what made how we worked and how our service was organised any different from, say, the child and family service next door.

The consensus reached after the usual animated discussion that characterised these meetings was that we worked from a feminist understanding

S. Egan, *Putting Feminism to Work*,
https://doi.org/10.1007/978-3-030-22109-6_1

of sexual violence. I was not entirely convinced. The child and family service next door, I countered, also seemed to have a feminist understanding of sexual violence but did not refer to themselves, nor did others refer to them, as a specifically 'feminist' service. The discussion turned to feminist 'values', which I possibly, a tad grumpily, found unsatisfactory, the latter being a concept that to this day makes my eyes glaze over; it always seems so vague. Someone suggested we take an unscheduled tea break to ponder the question further. I suspect that at this point I was probably trying people's patience, even as the still slightly indulged 'new kid on the block'.

We never did return to the question. This will not surprise anyone who has ever worked in such an organisation. The pressures of the work are constant. There are always issues and tasks that really cannot be set aside to make way for leisurely cerebral conversation: ensuring that a 24-hour crisis roster is covered; working with highly distressed survivors whose needs are critical and immediate; responding to calls from police and hospitals; running workshops in schools and community organisations; meeting with statutory child protection authorities; rushing out the door to pick up a child for their counselling appointment. There is very little downtime. Indeed, something that struck me when I returned to university to undertake my doctoral research was the quietude and orderliness, relatively speaking, of the academic work environment. I relished the luxury of having the space and time just to think.[1]

In retrospect, I would say that part of my difficulty in identifying specifically what made our service a feminist service (beyond a statement of fact) was that the 'typical' markers of a feminist service were missing. Management committees had replaced the earlier non-hierarchical collective structure, all services had a designated coordinator or manager and the era of women working in services based on their lived experience of sexual violence had ended.[2] I wanted to understand and to be able to 'see'

[1] I am of course not the first to make such an observation. Walker (2002), for example, makes a similar observation in relation to her work as a social worker and then academic in the U.K. I should also point out that I am reflecting here on my experiences as a doctoral researcher, which, despite the many real stressors of that role, does not entail the grind of 'workload points' or quite the same avalanche of 'administrative duties' that characterise the life of the contemporary 'fully fledged' academic.

[2] The other part of the problem was the unspoken—and at times spoken—assumption that the 1970s and 1980s represented the golden era of feminism, an era against which we would always find ourselves lacking. This, at times, played out as an unhelpful set of generation-based conflicts that I experienced as a worker in an individual service and within some of the

how feminist, or indeed other, ideas were evident in the mundane everyday practices and minutiae of regulatory decisions that collectively form a 'service' (for example, decisions about who can or cannot use a service).

In formulating these musings into the formal research questions that guided my empirical postdoctoral research, I found Michel Foucault's approach to knowledge and discourse provided the methodological tools I needed. Discourse, in the Foucauldian sense, is not solely about language but is evident in language, social practices and institutional regulations (Gavey, 2005, p. 346; Hall, 2004, p. 346). For example, we can find it in the discursive production of the desire to be 'a good mother' and the material and political effects that flow from that, including things like 'childcare books, hospital visits, routine check ups and the normalizing techniques that define satisfactory maternal health or development and so on' (Henriques, Hollway, Urwin, Venn, & Walkerdine, 1984, p. 219). Discourse governs the way a topic can be talked about and how ideas are put into practice, and it rules out or limits other ways of knowing. Discourses that have assumed dominance can be difficult to identify. They often appear natural or commonplace: the accepted way of thinking, doing and being.

During those first years in the field, I also began to question some of the comfortable dichotomies in which I had been so well schooled in the academy—at least within my particular location in the academy. The easy distinction between, for example, the ways medicine and psychiatry 'labelled' women through their diagnostic categories (as hysterical, depressed, frigid, borderline personality disorder [BPD]) as opposed to the liberatory 'naming' by feminism of women's previously unrecognised experiences of violence (as victims of sexual violence, domestic violence, or survivors of child sexual assault) did not always seem so clear cut. It seemed to me that we could also use these latter concepts and their attendant language to 'label', to assign a set of identifying characteristics or indeed an identity. The concept of being a 'survivor' or a 'victim' of sexual violence can function as a shorthand way of summing up a person and their experiences, of thinking we know who they are and the source of their worries and concerns or their strengths.

These sorts of musings remained largely private. They were not questions that I could have brought up at a team meeting. We were resolutely,

broader sector work with which I was involved—for example, when organising local Reclaim the Night marches.

almost stridently, anti-medical model. Concerns were regularly expressed, often in passing, about the increasing 'medicalisation' of sexual assault. To be honest, had I been questioned too closely, I am not sure I could have explained in any detail what the medicalisation of sexual assault actually was. Part of the problem of this inarticulacy was that certain terms had become embedded in polarised disciplinary, institutional and professional domains. Sometimes hurled almost as terms of abuse, they had come to signify little more than whose side you were on in whatever 'war' was being waged. The reductive language used to describe the perceived adversarial relationship between feminism and medicine troubled me.[3] It stymies the capacity for uncertainty or to query one's own position. I wanted more space for uncertainty and curiosity and to engage in dialogue. These initial thoughts about how feminist and medical knowledges function in practice are not always so clear cut enabled me to formulate what became a key research question in my empirical study. I became interested in investigating how trauma, a form of knowledge based in medicine and psychiatry, has been taken up in feminist work against sexual violence. Adopting a Foucauldian approach to discourse and knowledge production, I sought to understand *how* what appeared to be, and are often promoted as, two seemingly disparate forms of knowledge work together. I was interested in exploring their compatibility more than their incompatibility.

Overview, Context and Key Arguments

This book represents my attempt to respond to those questions and apparent contradictions that I had begun to formulate in those early experiences of practice and which I pursued through my doctoral research in the New South Wales (NSW) sexual assault services sector. It charts the development and application of feminist theories of sexual violence and trauma in

[3] On my return to university as a doctoral researcher, I did not necessarily find any more dialogic space to think through these questions. The only real difference at times seemed to be that the term had shifted to 'bio-medical model'. A turning point for me happened at a feminist conference in Australia. Presenting confidently about the dichotomisation of feminist and medical knowledges of sexual violence, I had noticed someone in the audience frowning and looking puzzled. During question time, she asked me on what basis I was discussing this dichotomy given the extent to which feminism has drawn on medical knowledges. Jennifer Germon's (2009) research, for example, highlights the origins of the concept of gender in the work of medical researchers such as John Money.

the sexual assault services sector in Australia. The key research question that frames the book is, what kind of feminist knowledge is built into the sexual assault services sector and how is it put to work? The book mounts two key arguments. First, I engage with a dominant contention within current feminist theory that state-sponsored institutional responses to sexual violence are restricted in what they can do to achieve feminist goals and have therefore left feminism behind. In the face of such elegiac narratives, I argue for recognition of the legitimacy of institutionalised feminism as an important component of feminist efforts to challenge and respond to sexual violence. In effect, I argue that although they are important in mobilising support for social change, grassroots movements on their own are not enough to tackle the complex problem of sexual violence embedded in the various patriarchal social institutions that support and sustain it. This book thus attempts to reconsider the value of institution-led responses against claims that subversive political action outside the apparatuses of the state is the only way to develop feminist knowledge, practices and interventions that can achieve social change.

Second, the book responds to a key criticism that sexual assault services, and feminist practitioners more broadly, rely on and reproduce a theory of trauma that places victims in an unhelpful position of helplessness and dependency. While I concur with existing scholarship that there are some problematic effects of the contemporary constructions of sexual victimhood as trauma, I suggest that this is the consequence of limitations or gaps in feminist theoretical work on sexual violence, rather than a problem endemic or specific to the process of institutionalisation of sexual assault services. Indeed despite these concerns there has been little empirical research by feminist scholars that has investigated the extent to which these concerns have come to fruition in the work of sexual assault services or feminist practitioners.

I argue that trauma theory is useful for the intimate and important emotional work that sexual assault counsellors do with their clients, whom they see when they are at their most vulnerable. This must be counterbalanced with the criticism that an emphasis on counselling and a reliance on knowledge based in psychiatry and clinical psychology merely reduces the social problem of sexual violence to a problem of individual healing. I argue in this book for a more complex understanding of the relationship between bodies, emotions and institutions as these connections are lived out in people's lives. In addressing this question of trauma, feminism and gendered violence, I suggest that the way in which the field works with the neurobiology of trauma may well be instructive for feminist scholarship on sexual violence. This book thus attends to the productive ways that feminist knowledge works through institutional settings where sexual assault workers come up against the effects of gendered violence on a daily basis.

The empirical work on which this book draws is as I have stated based on research conducted on Australian sexual assault services. Australia has been something of an 'early adopter' of institutionalised form of sexual assault and rape crisis service. The development of community based grass roots rape crisis centres and government sexual assault services (such as those based in hospitals for example) often occurred in tandem typically in the late 1970s and 1980s. Indeed the roll out of government sexual assault services across the state of NSW in the mid-1980s occurred at the same as the provision of funding to grassroots based incest centres that now form the non-government (NGO) sector child sexual assault services (Breckenridge, 1992; Carmody, 1995; Sawer, 1990). Moreover while rape crisis centres often began as unfunded grassroots based feminist responses the provision of government funding typically occurred relatively soon afterwards. For example the Sydney Rape Crisis Centre had begun to receive some government funding as early as 1974 (Carmody, 1995). As a consequence the trend towards a degree of integration into government (e.g. via the types of regulatory oversight that comes with receipt of government funding) is a long-standing feature of the Australian sexual assault services sector. In nations such as the UK and the USA widespread introduction of government services and government funding of the grassroots rape crisis centres is a more recent phenomenon. For example until the late 1990s the voluntary sector Rape Crisis Centres (RCC) that had emerged from the grassroots feminist movement were the primary means of specialist support for survivors of sexual assault in England and Wales. The provision of government based services Sexual Assault Referral Centres (primarily through statutory health sector), is relatively recent dating primarily from the early 2000s are a government led initiative and primarily a response to poor outcomes in criminal cases and subsequent negative attention given to criminal justice agencies (Hester & Lilley, 2017; Robinson & Hudson, 2011).

Yet while there are variations in specific service models adopted, in the local contexts such as specific incidents or events that precipitated their development there are overarching themes that accompany integration of services and responses into state apparatus. These include a move toward collaboration with systems such as police, medical, health systems and professionals systems, increased regulatory oversight by government, recruitment of workers from professions such as social work and psychology rather than via a grassroots feminist constituency and a disinclination by at least some services to explicitly identity as feminist services Moreover, as I lay out in Chapter 2 research that has focused on the influence and place of feminism in contemporary sexual assault services in places such as the United Kingdom (UK) and United States (US) has been informed by an understanding that feminism is about protest and grass roots activism and the adoption of an explicitly feminist identity by both services and practitioners. Moreover, perhaps because the roll out of government sexual assault service is more recent this research has focused on the effects of institutionalisation on the non-government rape crisis centres. One of my key aims in undertaking my research was to take a different approach to the place of feminism in contemporary sexual assault service by approaching feminism as a form of knowledge rather than as an identity (we are feminist services) or as defined through certain forms of political activity. Through doing so I aim to show the potential this type of approach has in illuminating the authority and indeed centrality of feminism in the makeup of contemporary sexual assault services. As Sylvia Walby (2011) notes in *The Future of feminism* (2011) feminism is no longer only an outsider protest movement but is increasingly entering mainstream organisations and institutions. An effect of this she argues is that significant aspects of contemporary feminism are not noticed precisely because they are less visible leading to the impression that 'feminism has faded away' (p. 52).

A Note on Terminology

Medicalisation

The term 'medicalisation' is often used to refer to the ways increasing numbers of everyday situations are brought under medical control and treated as medical problems (Conrad, 1992; Rose, 2007). Generally, the situation or problem is reframed as an illness or disorder, along with attendant medical language, the adoption of a medical framework to understand it, and a medical intervention to treat it. An example would be the way childbirth has changed from a natural event that took place in the woman's home to one that requires medical intervention, monitoring and routine hospitalisation. More recent examples include the menopause and problems with menstruation. Critics argue that doctors rather than patients benefit from medicalisation through increased power, money and control accrued individually and as a profession. Others, however, point to beneficial effects such as the way a medical diagnosis can reduce the stigma experienced by many individuals when their problem has not been recognised as having a medical basis (Broom & Woodward, 1996).

Broom and Woodward (1996) usefully distinguish between medicalisation, the increased scope of medicine, and medical dominance, which can occur at an individual level—when a doctor dominates a consultation—and at a policy level—when all the decision-makers are doctors and medical perspective and priorities determine the decisions made. As they point out, instances of medical dominance can occur equally in situations where the medical basis of the situation is uncontested, such as a person seeking treatment for a viral infection, as it can in situations where the legitimacy of medicalisation of the situation is contested.

However, 'medicalisation' is often used as a pejorative rather than a descriptive term. For example, it appears to have been first used in the social sciences literature in the 1960s to refer to the tendency of medical institutions to define non-conforming behaviours as illnesses and therefore as a way to manage the so-called deviant behaviour (Broom & Woodward, 1996).

Likewise, some of the most vocal early critics were those concerned with mental health (i.e. Szasz, 1963). Feminists in particular were vocal in drawing attention to the ways in which medicine pathologies normal female life events and to the poor treatment by psychiatrists of women with emotional difficulties and psychological distress (Chessler, 1972; Matthews, 1984). Medical definition and management of problems such as depression, which is diagnosed disproportionately in women, places the problem's source with the individual and limits interventions to those that focus on individual change rather than on the conditions in people's lives that cause their distress (Kirschner, 2013; Lafrance & McKenzie-Mohr, 2013; Marecek & Hare-Mustin, 2009). The framing of psychological distress as a disease, an illness or a disorder, it is argued, elides the role that the structural context of discrimination, oppression and exclusion plays in producing such distress.

The intensification of the medicalisation of emotional and psychological behaviour is typically identified as beginning with the sweeping changes made to the third edition of the *Diagnostic and Statistical Manual of*

Mental Disorders (DSM) in 1980.[4] By replacing the diffuse psychoanalytic concepts of DSM-II with their permeable boundaries between normal and abnormal, with specific diagnostic criteria and frameworks, DSM-III remodelled psychiatric nosology on a biomedical model in which increasingly specific descriptions and criteria are used to separate and identify different categories (Kirschner, 2013). Subsequent editions have resulted in the diffusion of deficit through increased quantity of diagnoses and lowered thresholds through the introduction of spectrums so that conditions can range from severe to mild (Kirschner, 2013).

The way in which the term medicalisation is used in relation to sexual assault varies. It can be used to critique the framing of the perpetration of sexual abuse as a type of psychiatric condition (Tosh, 2011). For example, paedophilia (paedophilic disorder) and exposing the genitals (exhibitionist disorder) are both included as psychiatric disorders in DSM-5 (American Psychiatric Association, 2013). It can also be used in relation to the medical examination conducted to gather physical evidence of the sexual assault and the weight given to that evidence and the evidence of medical experts as opposed to the victim's experience in the criminal legal process (Doe, 2012).

However, increasingly, medicalisation has come to denote feminist concern about the dominance of psychological trauma via the diagnosis of post-traumatic stress disorder (PTSD) as the primary way of understanding and responding to the problem of sexual violence (Lamb, 1999; Marecek, 1999; Peters, 2019; Warner & Wilkins, 2003). Echoing the more general critiques of the medicalisation of women's distress, concern focuses on the way the imposition of diagnostic frameworks, tools and techniques cast survivors' reactions as deficits that require treatment in order to be 'fixed'. PTSD 'individualises the problem so that survivors are held accountable for their recovery, and societal forces contributing to sexual violence are ignored (Peters, 2019, p. 77).

'Victims Versus 'Survivors'

I recognise that in the feminist community, the term 'survivor' is often preferred to 'victim' because the latter may be regarded as depriving

[4] Kirschner suggests psychoanalysis is an antecedent to medicalisation given that it frames all types of problems as amendable to psychiatric treatment and therefore increases the numbers of persons as possible patients.

women of agency. The term 'survivor' is typically used to emphasize and acknowledge the strength and resilience required to survive the ordeal of sexual violence. (Kelly, 1988; Kelly, Burton, & Regan, 1996), and to disrupt the negative associations that the term victim has with weakness, with 'passive suffering and interiority' (Mardorossian, 2014, p. 66), with fixing women's identity as wounded (Brown, 1995) and entrenching 'powerlessness as an identity' (Mardorossian, 2014, p. 66). However, concepts and terms can have unintended effects, sometimes being used interchangeably with the problematic term—in this case survivor—they were introduced to address (Alcoff & Gray, 1993; Gupta). Indeed Hunter (2010), found that almost half of her participants did not want to be identified as either victims or survivors of child sexual abuse because they did not want their identity linked to a particular childhood experience/s. That is, for these participants victim and survivor both had negative connotations because they were understood as imposing a predefined and all-encompassing identity. Cognisant of this Rape and Domestic Violence Services Australia [R&DVSA] (2018) elected to use neither term in a recent federal government submission on law reform. Rather they decided on 'the term people who have been impacted by sexual, family or domestic violence' and go onto explain that they do so 'in acknowledgement that, although experiences of violence are often very significant in a person's life, they nevertheless do not define that person' (p. 2).

However, while mindful of these debates I use both 'victim' and 'survivor' in this book for the sake of brevity and precision. I use 'victim' to indicate the experience of being the object of sexual violence and 'survivor' to indicate the subjective process of recovery from experiences of sexual violence. I do so cognisant that they exist on a continuum rather than as polarized opposites and that for some neither are terms which they identify or feel adequately captures their experiences (Hunter, 2010; R&DVSA, 2018). So through this book I speak of harm, of victimising experiences, of victims and survivors of sexual violence but I do so aware that people identities, categories and labels are always partial and never adequately sum up the entirety of an person or their experiences.

Common Terms Used in the Australian Field of Sexual Assault Service Provision

There are a number of terms that are used within and in the literature published about Australian sexual assault services with which not all readers may not be familiar. Terms such as sexual assault practitioners, sexual assault counsellors, and sexual assault workers are generally used interchangeably to refer to those employed in sexual assault services. Most services distinguish between these roles and that of the service manager or co-ordinator (again these terms are used interchangeably) although in many instances the service manager is also involved in counselling or other service responses such as community education. Terms such as 'the field of sexual assault service provision' or 'the field of sexual assault' reflect the professionalised nature of contemporary Australian services. For example the Australian Association of Social Workers (2020) uses the term 'fields of practice' to refer to the key areas in which social workers are employed. Child protection, domestic violence, drug and alcohol, health, youth and sexual assault are all considered fields of practice. Within a given field of practice one could be employed in a number of different capacities for example as a caseworker or counsellor, as a manager, a policy analyst or researcher or as a community educator. Consequently the 'field of sexual assault service provision' refers to the network of individual services and the types of work undertaken in those services as well as to the committees, peak bodies, training organisations and policy analyst positions that together make up this field.

Chapter Overview

The first part of Chapter 2 outlines the key concerns feminist scholars have raised about the place of feminism in contemporary work against sexual violence, before moving on to an overview of the Foucauldian feminist approach to knowledge production that frames the book. In the remainder of the chapter, I provide an overview of the research I conducted in a local Australian field of sexual assault service provision, which acts as a case study throughout the book. Chapter 3 begins by locating contemporary feminist knowledge/s of sexual assault in historical context by providing a brief historical overview of popular and professional representations of rape from the late-nineteenth century onwards. I use these representations as juxtapositions with which to illuminate the different understandings feminist analyses have brought to bear on the question of 'what sexual assault is' and the different ways this enables us to respond. Using my empirical work as an example, I illustrate the ways these key feminist ideas enable the basic rules of engagement or policies and practices that underpin sexual assault services. Through doing so, I aim to make visible what feminism 'look like' when it operates through service structures and regulatory frameworks and is put to work through individual interventions with victims and survivors. Far from dissipating or being in decline, I suggest that feminist knowledge holds an authoritative, almost naturalised, position in the contemporary NSW field of sexual assault service provision.

Chapters 4 and 5 examine the way trauma has been produced as a feminist knowledge and practice in the field of sexual assault service provision. I re-engage with the feminist concerns about the dominance of trauma, particularly the incursions of diagnostic frameworks associated with medicine and psychiatry outlined in Chapter 2, and draw on my empirical research to argue that trauma is not necessarily tied in any *essential* way to psychiatric pathology but can be put to work productively as part of contemporary feminist practice. I draw on interviews with sexual assault workers to illuminate what the deployment of trauma looks like 'in practice' and to examine the possibilities and the problems posed by this uptake. The question of the epistemological status of trauma as medical and psychiatric knowledge is, I suggest, less pertinent to the terms of the debate than its potential in enabling practitioners to recognise, understand and assist victims with the material and bodily effects of violence. In particular, I highlight the productive ways practitioners integrate neurobiological understandings of trauma into their work. The final chapter (Chapter 6) considers the possibilities that this uptake of neurobiology in practice may suggest for reintroducing the (biological) body into feminist analyses of sexual violence before concluding with a brief revisiting of the 'perils' of institutionalisation thesis in light of the authority, visibility and robustness of feminist knowledges and practices demonstrated through the body of the book.

In summary, the book brings together theory and practice to reconsider the contribution of state-based sexual violence services to feminist knowledges and aspirations. The empirical research on which it draws provides a basis from which to problematise the ways the terms of the debates have been framed and to bring a different perspective to bear on issues such as the uptake of neurobiological approaches to trauma in applied feminist work on sexual violence. Finally, the extent to which the book draws on empirical research undertaken in an applied field represents an important intervention into feminist scholarship and debates on violence against women.

References

Alcoff, L., & Gray, A. (1993). Survivor discourse: Transgression or recuperation? *Signs, 18*(2), 260–290.

American Psychiatric Association. (2013). *Diagnostic and statistical manual of mental disorders: DSM-5* (5th ed.). Washington, DC: Author.

Australian Association of Social Workers (AASW). (2020). Fields of practice. Retrieved from https://www.aasw.asn.au/professional-development/fields-of-practice

Breckenridge, J. (1992). An exotic phenomenon? Incest and child rape. In J. Breckenridge & M. Carmody (Eds.), *Crimes of violence: Australian responses to rape and child sexual assault* (pp. 18–37). Sydney, Australia: Allen & Unwin.

Broom, D. H., & Woodward, R. V. (1996). Medicalisation reconsidered: Toward a collaborative approach to care., *18*(3), 357–378. https://doi.org/10.1111/1467-9566.ep10934730

Brown, W. (1995). *States of injury: Power and freedom in late modernity.* Princeton, NJ: Princeton University Press.

Carmody, M. (1995). *Site of struggle: The development of sexual assault services in New South Wales, Australia* (Unpublished doctoral dissertation). University of New South Wales, Australia.

Chessler, P. (1972). *Women and madness.* New York, NY: Avon Books.

Conrad, P. (1992). Medicalization and social control. *Annual Review of Sociology, 18*, 209–232.

Doe, J. (2012). Who benefits from the sexual assault evidence kit? In E. A. Sheehy (Ed.), *Sexual assault in Canada: Law, legal practice and women's activism.* Ottowa, Canada: University of Ottawa Press.

Gavey, N. (2005). *Just sex? The cultural scaffolding of rape.* London, UK: Routledge.

Germon, J. (2009). *Gender: A genealogy of an idea.* New York, NY: Palgrave Macmillan.

Hall, S. (2004). Foucault and discourse. In C. Seale (Ed.), *Social research methods reader* (pp. 345–349). London, UK: Routledge.

Henriques, H., Hollway, W., Urwin, C., Venn, C., & Walkerdine, V. (1984). *Changing the subject: Psychology, social regulation and subjectivity.* New York, NY and London, UK: Methuen.

Hester, M., & Lilley, S.-J. (2017). More than support to court: Rape victims and specialist sexual violence services. *International Review of Victimology, 24*(3), 313–328. https://doi.org/10.1177/0269758017742717

Hunter, S. V. (2010). Evolving narratives about childhood sexual abuse: Challenging the dominance of the victim and survivor paradigm. *The Australian and New Zealand Journal of Family Therapy, 31*, 176–198. https://doi.org/10.1375/anft.31.2.176

Kelly, L. (1988). *Surviving sexual violence.* Oxford, UK: Polity.

Kelly, L., Burton, S., & Regan, L. (1996). Beyond victim or survivor: Sexual violence, identity and feminist theory and practice. In L. Adkins & V. Merchant (Eds.), *Sexualizing the social explorations in sociology* (pp. 71–101). London, UK: Palgrave Macmillan.

Kirschner, S. R. (2013). Diagnosis and its discontents: Critical perspectives on psychiatric nosology and the DSM. *Feminism & Psychology, 23*(1), 10–28. https://doi.org/10.1177/0959353512467963

Lafrance, M. N., & McKenzie-Mohr, S. (2013). The DSM and its lure of legitimacy. *Feminism & Psychology, 23*(1), 119–140. https://doi.org/10.1177/0959353512467974

Lamb, S. (1999). Constructing the victim: Popular images and lasting labels. In S. Lamb (Ed.), *New versions of victims. Feminists struggle with the concept* (pp. 108–138). New York, NY and London, UK: New York University Press.

Mardorossian, C. M. (2014). *Framing the rape victim: Gender and agency reconsidered.* New Brunswick, NJ: Rutgers University Press.

Marecek, J. (1999). Trauma talk in feminist clinical practice. In S. Lamb (Ed.), *New versions of victims: Feminist struggle with the concept* (pp. 158–182). New York, NY: New York University Press.

Marecek, J., & Hare-Mustin, R. T. (2009). Clinical psychology: The politics of madness. In *Critical psychology: An introduction* (2nd ed., pp. 75–92). Thousand Oaks, CA: Sage Publications Ltd.

Matthews, J. J. (1984). *Good and mad women: The historical construction of femininity in twentieth-century Australia.* Sydney, Australia: Allen & Unwin.

Peters, S. M. (2019). Demedicalizing the aftermath of sexual assault: Toward a radical humanistic approach. *Journal of Humanistic Psychology*, 1–23. Online. https://doi.org/10.1177/0022167819831526

Rape and Domestic Violence Services Australia (R&DVSA). (2018). Submission to NSW Law Reform Commission. Consent in relation to sexual offences. 29 June 2018 Retrieved from www.rape-dvservices.org.au/uploads/main/PDFs/Legal-submissions/RDVSA-Submission-Review-of-Consent-Law-Website.pdf

Robinson, A., & Hudson, K. (2011). Different yet complementary: Two approaches to supporting victims of sexual violence in the UK. *Criminology & Criminal Justice, 11*(5), 515–533. https://doi.org/10.1177/1748895811419972

Rose, N. (2007). Beyond medicalisation. *Lancet, 369*, 700–702. https://doi.org/10.1016/S01406736(07)60319-5

Sawer, M. (1990). *Sisters in suits. Women and public policy in Australia.* North Sydney, Australia: Allen & Unwin.

Szasz, T. (1963). *Law, liberty and psychiatry.* New York, NY: Macmillan.

Tosh, J. (2011). The medicalisation of rape? A discursive analysis of 'paraphilic coercive disorder' and the psychiatrization of sexuality. *Psychology of Women Section Review, 13*, 2–12.

Walby, S. (2011). *The future of feminism*. Cambridge, UK: Polity Press.
Walker, H. (2002). *A genealogy of equality: The curriculum for social work education and training*. London, UK: Woburn Press.
Warner, S., & Wilkins, T. (2003). Diagnosing distress and reproducing disorder: Women, child sexual abuse and 'borderline personality disorder'. In P. Reavey & S. Warner (Eds.), *New feminist stories of child sexual abuse: Sexual scripts and dangerous dialogues* (pp. 167–186). London, UK: Routledge.

CHAPTER 2

Surveying the Landscape: Histories, Context and Contemporary Issues

Introduction

Through this book, I enter into a dialogue with contemporary feminist debate about the place of feminism in contemporary work against sexual violence and aim to provide an alternative to the dominant narrative of decline and co-option. In the current chapter, I engage with scholarly concerns about the diminution of feminism by introducing the reader to the methodological rationale for my empirical study on the production of feminist knowledge in sexual assault services in the state of NSW, Australia. The case study provides the crucial foundation for the argument in this book—that what has come to constitute feminist knowledge in the sexual assault services sector ought to be treated as a serious object of empiricist enquiry and an active production, rather than an inert fact. In this chapter, I explain the methodological approach used to design and conduct the study to show how the sexual assault services sector operates as a historically situated 'field of feminist practice'. This exploration provides a broad account of the development of sexual assault support organisations in NSW as feminist women's services, including personal narratives by

This chapter contains material reprinted from *Women's Studies International Forum*, 74(May–June), Suzanne Egan, "Excavating feminist knowledges and practices in the field of sexual assault service provision: An Australian case study", 169–178, Copyright (2019), with permission from Elsevier.

S. Egan, *Putting Feminism to Work*,
https://doi.org/10.1007/978-3-030-22109-6_2

women who worked in and were part of the sector's early development. The chapter concludes with an outline of the current structure of NSW sexual assault services and synopsis of the constitution and operation of feminist knowledge across these services.

Contemporary Debates

Feminism has had a profound influence on public recognition of and political responses to the issue of violence against women. Indeed, politicisation of sexual violence is often understood as one of the key drivers of the second-wave feminist movement that arose in Western countries in the 1970s and 1980s. Feminists were instrumental in campaigning to bring the issue of violence against women to community attention, mounting sustained political protests against poor treatment by medical, police and legal systems, mobilising to provide direct support for victims and undertaking research that documented the nature and extent of violence against women (Breckenridge, 1992; Carmody, 1992; Genovese, 2000; Irwin & Thorpe, 1996; Jones & Cook, 2008; Weeks & Gilmore, 1996; Whittier, 2009). The rape crisis centres set up and run by feminists played a key role in providing a woman-centred and safe environment for victims and working to achieve the widespread social and political changes needed to prevent sexual violence. However, while the origins of what is now a formalised sector of sexual assault policy, practice and service provision in the women's movement is widely acknowledged (Breckenridge, 1992; Carmody, 1995; Spongberg, 1998; Weeks & Gilmore, 1996), there has been growing disquiet about the continued strength and influence of feminism.

Feminist scholars have questioned the place of feminism in contemporary work against sexual violence, raising concerns about what Beres, Crow, and Gotell (2009) call the 'perils' of institutionalisation. This refers to the extent to which government or philanthropic funding of rape crisis and sexual assault centres has resulted in a move away from political activism and social change towards a professionalised and depoliticised service-provider model (Beres et al., 2009; Corrigan, 2014; Jones & Cook, 2008; Maier, 2008; Mardorossian, 2002; Whalley & Hackett, 2017).[1]

[1] These types of concerns are reflective of those expressed about the institutionalisation of Anglo–American feminism more broadly within the academy, government and non-government sites (for examples of commentary, see Brown, 2003; Hemmings, 2005; Probyn, 1998).

Critics highlight the extent to which institutionalisation has resulted in a shift to collaborating with, rather protesting against, police, legal and medical systems that perpetuate gender inequality[2] (Campbell, Baker, & Mazurek, 1998; Maier, 2008; Whalley & Hackett, 2017). Campbell et al. (1998), for example, point out that while federal legislation in the United States increased the funding available to violence against women services, those that were funded were curtailed in their ability to protest against the government or be involved in political activism. Bumiller (2008) in particular has been critical of the overreliance of feminist anti-violence work in the United States on legal reform and criminal prosecution, arguing that this has had the effect of co-opting feminists into the 'law and order' agenda associated with the neoliberal state. For feminist critics, the incorporation of sexual assault organisations into the regulatory apparatus of government has dissipated from this sector, if not removed, the dedicated political activism that once drove demands for social change (Bumiller, 2008; Whittier, 2009). These types of changes have given scholars reason to query the extent to which sexual assault support organisations actually continue to identify as 'feminist' (Corrigan, 2014; Maier, 2008; Whalley & Hackett, 2017). Corrigan (2014), who interviewed advocates from more than 100 rape crisis centres across six U.S. states, found that many individuals and services did not identify as feminist. For some organisations and practitioners, this was a strategic decision based on concerns that publicly identifying as feminist would jeopardise their funding or have a negative effect on their relationships with the police and medical practitioners. Others did not identify as feminist because 'working from a social service and helping perspective they did not see any relationship between sexual assault and struggles for gender equity' (Corrigan, 2014, p. 281).

A concomitant concern centres on the increasing prioritisation of individual counselling and therapy using psychological approaches that focus on individual healing as the preferred way of responding to rape (Burstow, 2005; Cvetkovich, 2003; Lamb, 1999; Marecek, 1999; Wilkin & Hillock, 2014). Much of this critique focuses on the increasing dominance of psychological trauma—and associated diagnoses and treatment models—as

[2] For example, Whalley and Hackett (2017), in an ethnographic study of one U.S. rape crisis telephone line, found that advocates prioritised calls from police and hospitals over victims or other organisations and in training were told to question victims about their reasons if they did not want to make a report to police. According to the authors, these practices began when the local crisis telephone line was incorporated into a national hotline.

the accepted way of understanding and responding to sexual violence. Such approaches, it is argued, pathologise the 'normal' effects of sexual victimisation as symptoms to be 'fixed' and work against traditional feminist principles that promote strength, choice and autonomy (Burstow, 2005; Marecek, 1999; Wilkin & Hillock, 2014). Stark (2007), for example, argues that in the United States, this individualised approach has had the effect of foreclosing the politicisation of survivors and their capacity to mobilise to challenge patriarchy.

A number of these writers and researchers acknowledge a focus on suffering and psychological harm as having played an important role in feminist work against sexual violence: that is, in challenging discourses of silence and blame and in gaining public recognition of sexual violence as a serious social issue (e.g. Lamb, 1999; Mardorossian, 2002; O'Dell, 2003; Reavey, 2003; Reavey & Brown, 2007). However, there is concern about the problematic ways the 'harm' story (O'Dell, 2003) positions victims of sexual violence, depriving them of agency and placing them in a position of ongoing vulnerability. Sharon Lamb (1999) in *Constructing the Victim: Popular Images and Lasting Labels* argues that the dominance of 'trauma talk' has in effect reduced a moral and political issue to a mental health problem. In these accounts, the dominance of trauma in feminist work against sexual violence is typically attributed to a decline in feminism as a social movement and political force (Lamb, 1999; Mardorossian, 2002; Marecek, 1999; O'Dell, 2003; Whittier, 2009).

Marecek (1999, p. 165), in an example of this genre of work, suggests that the medicalisation of feminist practice is evident in the widespread attribution of a 'trauma' framework among feminist therapists to their clients' experiences of childhood sexual abuse. Based on interviews with feminist therapists working across a range of issues in the United States, she found that 'trauma talk' dominated the interview data, with participants typically identifying the problems that had initially brought their clients to therapy (the presenting problem) as symptomatic of the underlying problem of childhood trauma, usually child sexual assault.

To the therapists using a trauma framework, women's symptoms of distress could be understood as 'normal' responses to 'abnormal' or catastrophic events, rather than as symptomatic of an abnormality or pre-existing pathology (Marecek, 1999, pp. 162–163). Consequently, they view trauma as affirming a core tenet of feminism—that sexual abuse is not the victim's fault—and as distinctively different from the pathologising language and practices of medicine. Indeed, Marecek (1999) found that for some therapists, the trauma model had *become* feminist practice so that assessments of and interventions with all clients were based on the concept of underlying trauma. Pointing out that 'trauma' is a medical concept, she argues that its conceptual framework uses the same logic as psychopathology: specifically, that it works according to a simple 'cause and effect' explanation, which reduces women's experiences to a uniform set of symptoms (Marecek, 1999, p. 165). Marecek associates the dominance of 'trauma talk' among feminist therapists with a decline in feminist influence and the possibility that feminist therapists may 'consciously or unconsciously' have modelled their practices on high-status professions like medicine (Marecek, 1999, pp. 165–170).

Collectively, this scholarship points to the erosion of an explicitly feminist political agenda in the field of sexual assault through its entanglement with state-based bureaucracy, a marked shift towards professionalisation, and individualised interventions that approach sexual assault as an expression of psychologised harm. Essentially, feminist criticism of the contemporary field of sexual assault comes down to the perception that feminist work against sexual violence has been co-opted into a conservative political agenda that focuses on the effects of sexual violence at the expense of any sustained commitment to radically changing the structural gender inequalities that enable and support sexual assault.

The assumption running through much of this scholarship is that to be considered 'feminist', organisations and people who work against sexual violence do so through 'activist' strategies that aim to bring about broad-based social change. This equation of feminist work with social and political activism runs through the empirical work conducted in this area (e.g. Beres et al., 2009; Campbell et al., 1998; Jones & Cook, 2008; Maier, 2008). For example, Beres et al.'s (2009) influential Canadian study was designed to elicit evidence on the extent to which rape crisis centres continue to identity as feminist pro-women organisations that remain involved in anti-rape activism, such as political marches and campaigns, rather than just counselling services. Similarly, others (e.g. Corrigan, 2014; Maier, 2008; Whalley & Hackett, 2017) use criteria such as whether services explicitly identify as feminist (in mission statements or other written material) and whether they are involved in particular activities, such as political activism, to determine whether the service is feminist. In addition, as I noted in Chapter 1 perhaps due to their relatively recent development in the United Kingdom and United States little of this research has been extended to government or statutory sexual assault services but rather has focused on the non-government rape crisis centres that trace their origins to grassroots rape crisis movement.

It appears to me that these critiques are troublingly polarising in determining that service approaches to sexual assault must take place outside or only position themselves in opposition to state-based systems and institutions (law, medicine and government) to be adequately feminist. In the context of her work on the Indian women's movement, Srila Roy (2009, 2011) suggests that such critiques typically use as their point of nostalgic comparison the grassroots women's organisations of the 1970s and 1980s. The problem with this approach, she argues, is that the concept of a more politically 'authentic' past comes to function as the normative standard for the present, against which current organisations—with their professionalised workforce and government, or foreign-donor funding—can only ever be found wanting. Debates cleave into a series of temporally based binaries: the 'past is political, radical, "spontaneous" and "real", while the present is apolitical, professionalized, "careerist", and individualized' (Roy, 2009, p. 346). This very specific and particular interpretation of 'feminism' means that other forms of feminism remain invisible and, therefore, do not form part of current debates and concerns about the place, role and influence of feminism in contemporary work against sexual assault.

This concern led me to conduct empirical research on contemporary Australian sexual assault services. I wanted to learn more about the place of feminism in the contemporary sexual assault services setting and how feminist knowledges have been formed and transformed within the sector. To do so, I developed a project that investigated the production of feminist knowledge in the NSW sexual assault services sector, focusing largely on service delivery. The data I collected consisted of documents produced by and/or for these services and interviews with practitioners. Many of my interviewees clearly articulated the historical association between feminism and the field of sexual assault, which was typically a source of pride. In the words of one participant, they were 'a child of the feminist movement'. While they were clear that their ideas and practices came from feminism, some expressed concern that 'feminism seems to be talked about less and less', that 'feminism has gone underground' and has declined as a political movement. For a few practitioners, particularly those with lengthy working histories, this reflected the changes they had experienced in moving from collectives to services run by management committees, for example. For a number of other practitioners, though, the concern seemed to be based on a 'received history', the sort of account of 'how things used to be' that circulates through organisations, institutions and social movements. In this chapter, I revisit this project to suggest that these narratives do not need to be read as evidence that feminism in the sexual assault services sector has become diluted or corrupted, or no longer exists. Rather, I ask instead that we consider the different question of how feminist knowledge might be constituted and operationalised in these spaces.

In what follows, I lay out the types of research conducted on Australian sexual assault services to date, introduce the project and methodological approach used to design and conduct my empirical study of sexual assault services in NSW, Australia, and explain the historical development of the sexual assault services sector as a 'field of feminist practice'. This includes histories of feminist women's services, accounts produced by women who worked in and were part of the early development of services, and histories of the work of feminist bureaucrats. I also outline the current structure of NSW sexual assault services and the constitution and operation of feminist knowledge across these services and provide a synopsis of the key findings from the study.

Surveying the Research on Contemporary Australian Sexual Assault Services

While the foundational role of feminism in the development of Australian sexual assault services (e.g. Breckenridge, 1992; Burke 1992; Carmody, 1995; Wills, 2007, 2008) and influence on early practices, (Blyth & Vernan, 1992; Case, 1992; Cora, 1992; Freedman & Want, 1992; Laing, 1992; Members of the North Shore Women's Group with, Carmody, & Blyth, 1992)[3] is well documented, there is an absence of research on the relationship between feminism and the contemporary sexual assault services sector. Indeed, the knowledge produced about the contemporary field of sexual assault is characteristic of the type of knowledge typically produced about established sectors and fields of service provision. Broadly, this can be referred to as evaluative or evaluation research. The aim of this type of research is to map measure and evaluate the effectiveness of the

[3] The commentary on feminist practices was published in an edited collection of articles, *Crimes of violence: Australian responses to rape and child sexual assault*, by Breckenridge and Carmody (1992). Although it is titled 'Australian responses' most of the authors worked in the NSW sexual assault field in policy, practice and training positions.

services, practices, policies, systems and formalised responses, which together make up an institutionalised field of service provision. The aim is to identify gaps and measure effectiveness of already established responses rather than to politicise the given issue so as to establish the need for such responses (Fraser, 1989).

Characteristic research includes: “mapping” types of service provision (National Association of Services Against Sexual Violence, 2000; Olle, 2005) and access and equity practices (Weeks, 2002); codifying standards of practice (Carmody et al., 2009; Dean, Hardiman, & Draper, 1998); reports about the effectiveness of the systems, such as the legal and health systems, that respond to sexual assault victims (Attorney General’s Department. New South Wales, 2006; Bluett-Boyd, 2014; Breckenridge, Rees, Valentine, & Murray, 2016; Leviore, 2005; NSW Violence Against Women Specialist Unit, 2006; Olle, 2005); and identification of additional fields in which a response to sexual assault is either absent or inadequate. Included in the latter are mental health services (Murray & Powell, 2008; Watson, Maylea, Roberts, Hill, & McCallum, 2020), domestic violence (Heenan, 2004; Keel, Fergus, & Heenan, 2005) and drug and alcohol services (Quadara, Stathopoulos, & Jenkinson, 2015, and organisations that assist women trafficked for sexual exploitation (Fergus, 2005). Research literature about populations serviced by the sector focuses on gaps in and barriers to service provision for particular types of sexual assault victims. These include adults sexually abused in childhood (Fergus & Keel, 2005; Neame & Heenan, 2004; Olle, 2005), male victims (Crome, 2006), trafficked women (Fergus, 2005), Indigenous victims (Blagg, Bluett-Boyd, & Williams, 2015; Cox, 2008; Keel et al., 2005), victims who live with disabilities (Frawley, Dyson, Robinson, & Dixon, 2015; Keel et al., 2005; Murray & Powell, 2008) and victims from culturally and linguistically diverse backgrounds (Lay, 2006; Mitra-Kahn, Newbigin, & Hardefeldt, 2016).

The most recent attention to the place of feminism in the Australian field of sexual assault is a complication of articles *Challenging Silence: Innovative responses to sexual and domestic violence*, edited by Breckenridge and Laing in 1999. Running through the collection, which contains commentary and reflection by Australian practitioners, policy makers and researchers is concern that the gains made by feminists during the 1970s and 1980s are under threat and the influence of feminism is in decline. Issues explored include silencing practices such as professional discourses that relegate the voices of victims to the margins of credible knowledge

(Breckenridge, 1999), structures that deny women's experiences of abuse, including the legal system (Doyle & Barbato, 1999) and mental health systems (Davidson & McNamara, 1999).[4]

A Feminist Foucauldian Approach to Knowledge Production

Feminist engagement with Foucault's work has been extensive, spanning almost three decades. Sawicki (2005), in a review of the reception of Foucault's work in Anglo-American feminist scholarship, usefully highlights key areas of convergence between his writing and feminist concerns. She emphasises the overlap between feminist concerns with the politics of everyday life and forms of social control associated with the human sciences and related institutions, and Foucault's concept of modern power as operating outside the formal state apparatus, through practices and regulatory techniques associated with the human sciences. Early feminist Foucauldian scholars, such as Bartky (1988) and Bordo (1988, 1993), used Foucault's concept of power to theorise contemporary practices of femininity, arguing that modern patriarchal power operates through the normalising processes—for example, the fitness regimes, dietary practices, clothing and hairstyles—that produce recognisably feminine bodies. Feminists writing on sexual and gender identity have drawn extensively on Foucault's theorisation of homosexuality as a socially and historically constructed category of personhood. Judith Butler (1990, 1993) exemplified this genre of work, extending Foucault's work on the historical and thoroughly modern construction of the homosexual subject to argue that gendered identities and subject positions such as *female/male* and *woman/man* are similarly socially produced rather than fixed categories (Deveaux, 1994; Sawicki, 2005).

Foucault problematised received truths about different categories of people—the mad, the criminal and the sexually deviant—and questioned the inevitability of the accepted practices with such people. He did so by undertaking meticulously detailed historical research using his unique methodological tools and analytical concepts. These studies aimed to

[4] This type of positioning of feminism as under threat or in decline was part of a more generalised wave of concern about a backlash against feminism in Australian social policy and political life during the 1990's and early 2000s (see for example Phillips, 2006; Schofield & Goodwin, 2006).

question the certainty about practices and institutional arrangements often presented as having no alternative: that it was inevitable asylums would be set up to treat the mentally ill, that criminals would be imprisoned and that sexual freedom could only be attained by discovering and accepting one's sexual orientation (Gutting, 2005a, p. 10). For example, in *The Will to Knowledge* (1998), Foucault argues that although there is a long history of human beings engaging in homosexual acts, homosexuality as an identity, a subject position or a discernible category of personhood has a relatively short history. The 'homosexual', he suggests, is a modern identity category, the product of the nineteenth-century sciences that codified sexuality and of the modern practices of assessment, observation and monitoring associated with the control of sexuality that had formed sexuality as an object of scientific scrutiny. Such practices, he points out, are enacted both by others (the psychiatrists who conduct assessments) and by the subjects themselves who, as they come to know themselves via these practices, are able to assess and monitor themselves as self-forming subjects.

However, to approach subject positions—such as the homosexual, the psychiatric patient or the survivor of sexual violence—does not mean denying the existence of madness or mental illness, or questioning the reality of the experience and effect of mental illness. As Foucault emphasised,

> When I say that I am studying the 'problematization' of madness, crime, or sexuality, it is not a way of denying the reality of such phenomena. On the contrary, I have tried to show that it was precisely some real existent in the world which was the target of social regulation at a given moment. (Foucault, 2001, p. 171)

A Foucauldian enquiry into knowledge production is not an investigation into whether ideas, beliefs or theories about a given problem *are* 'true', but is, rather, an enquiry into *how* the problem or topic of analysis has been constituted. An underlying premise is that each society, discipline and domain of knowledge production has its own accepted truths or the type of knowledge or discourses that it finds acceptable and promotes. This regime includes mechanisms for distinguishing truth from falseness, the means used to sanction discourse, the procedures that are given value in pursuing truth and the status of those positioned as speaking this 'truth' (Foucault, 1980a). Although feminists have always engaged in critical debate over the 'truth' position of other (masculinist) forms of knowledge, it has not been conventional for feminists to consider feminism as a 'regime of truth' (Bell, 1993).

An effect of adopting a Foucauldian position or theory of knowledge is that feminism, too, is approached as a form of knowledge with its own regime of truth, its own mechanisms and procedures for pursuing truth, for sanctioning some discourses but not others and for the positioning of those accorded the status of speaking that truth. Engagement with a Foucauldian approach to knowledge production means recognising that in some problematisations or topics of inquiry, feminism may have assumed the status of 'truth' and achieved the sort of dominance more usually associated with (patriarchal) knowledge/s that has/have been the object of feminist critique.

Indeed, Bell (1993, p. 175) argues persuasively that in her own discipline of sociology, feminism 'has won' the discursive battle over incest. As she notes, incest has long been a topic of interest to social scientists, sociologists and social anthropologists as an example of a universal social rule, 'the incest prohibition'. It is now understood, for example, that discussions of incest are meant to address questions of sexual violence rather than the origin and function of the incest taboo. As she so aptly comments,

> Incest is a topic of long standing interest to social scientists. Over the course of a century or so, sociologists and social anthropologists have explored the incest prohibition as the example *par excellence* of a social rule. Many influential social scientists contributed to the debates around the prohibition of incest. Initially, the questions posed reflected the dominant sociological interest in finding social facts and order in life. The incest prohibition was declared a safe fact, a universal social rule, and debates took this as a point of departure, asking either 'how did the incest prohibition originate?' or 'why did societies institute such a taboo, i.e. what function does it serve?' In these discussions, the actual occurrence of incest was considered rare and where acknowledged it was considered outside the remit of sociology, inhabiting instead the realms of abnormal psychology, where it did not contradict the sorts of questions under investigation. If sociology's task was to uncover the broad social patterns of life, it was not those who committed incest who were the focus of attention, but the majority who did not. Those who commit incest do not threaten the notion of the incest prohibition as a fundamental social rule because they are regarded not as *social* beings, but as 'misfits'. (Bell, 1993, pp. 1–2, italics in original)

The 'discovery' of incest as a widespread practice rather than a rare crime has meant incest is no longer understood within sociology as a social rule requiring explanation but as a social problem to be uncovered and measured. However, Bell (1993) points out that in the move from the prohibition to the practice, 'theory does not somehow get left behind' (p. 22). Surveys need to be devised and data interpreted and discussed, all of which requires some form of theorising. She argues that feminism has been predominant in taking up the challenge of asking sociological questions and in providing alternatives to individualistic explanations of the widespread practice of incest. Second-wave feminists argued that incest was a form of sexual abuse, and their analyses positioned incest as a form of male violence that occurs in a society in which men are able to exert control over women and children. Thus, incest came to be located within the model of the feminist analysis of rape, a conceptual and political relocation reflected in the renaming of incest from 'father–daughter incest' (Herman, 1981) to 'father–daughter rape' (Ward, 1984) and 'incestuous assault' (S. Butler, 1985).

Through examination of incestuous abuse as a social issue, feminists point to the normality rather than the abnormality of offenders and argue that understood in the context of the power dynamics and normative understandings of sexuality in patriarchal society, the practice of incest should not surprise. Indeed, Bell (1993) argues that feminism

> presents, even if in the margins of feminist texts and discussions, a profound *theoretical* shift in the way in which incest is conceived in the sociological imagination ... Feminists argue that incest cannot be regarded as *asocial* at all, but has to be analysed instead in direct relation to the social structures, which are continually produced and reproduced as 'normal'. Turning the earlier sociological discussions on their head, therefore, feminists argue that it is not the incest prohibition but, rather, the actual occurrence of incest, which provides a key to sociological understanding of social structure and culture. (p. 33, italics in original)

Thus, feminist knowledge of incest can be understood as having achieved the position of 'truth' in the discipline of sociology and in doing so has had a profound impact on the question of 'what is sociology and sociological inquiry'. Through the use of the Foucauldian concepts of knowledge, power and truth, Bell illuminates both the impact and the specificity of that impact. The relocation of the practice of incest from one field of disciplinary inquiry to another (abnormal psychology to sociology) has led to the production of a new object of sociological analysis (the practice rather than the taboo of incest) and to profound change in sociological understandings of 'social facts' and broader social patterns and structures.

Similarly Nicola Gavey (2019) provides a persuasive account of the influence that feminist analysis have had on social sciences research on the now burgeoning field of social sciences research into the prevalence, causes and effects of sexual violence. As Gavey points out rape was an issue that until the advent of the second wave women's movement attracted little interest in the social sciences; while the few studies that were conducted proceeded from the premise that victims were responsible for their abuse. Early pioneering early social science researchers such as Diana Russell, Mary Koss and Martha Burt were instrumental both in drawing the attention of the social sciences to the issue and in explicitly using feminist analyses of sexual assault to inform their studies. Burt, a psychologist, set out in the late 1970s to operationalise and test what she referred to as 'some of the tenets of feminist analyses of rape' as theorised by feminist such as Brownmiller and Griffin (Burt, 1980, p. 217). Informed by these analyses her study, published in mainstream experimental social psychology journal, the *Journal of Personality and Social Psychology* set out to examine the occurrence of rape supportive attitudes, or rape myths which she defined as false, prejudicial beliefs about rape, rape victims and rapists (Gavey, 2019).[5] Similarly Diana Russell (1982, 1984) who undertook the first US prevalence study incorporated feminist knowledge of sexual assault into her research design. For example cognisant that 'rape myths' might prevent participants willingness to disclose as well as their propensity to identify their experiences as rape, only one of the 38 interview questions used the word rape. Instead a range of open ended questions were asked about specific behaviours with different groups of men, and aware of the breadth of societal misconceptions the interviewers were given specific training about rape and incestuous abuse.

While often no longer be explicitly identified as feminist these types of insights, knowledge and analysis continue to inform social sciences research. For example Leviore (2005), in a review of sexual assault

[5] For example the majority of Burt's sample agreed with statements such as that the victim was promiscuous or had a bad reputation, that many rape reports were malicious and many believed acquaintance rape to be less serious than by a stranger.

prevalence studies refers to studies that use behaviourally specific questions and give participants multiple opportunities to disclose abuse, simply as 'good science'. Yet these are methods that little more than three decades ago Russell had devised by drawing on and incorporating feminist theorisation of sexual violence into her research design. Similarly, a multitude of proclivity studies have found that many 'normal' men report there are circumstances in which they would force a woman to have sex. As Gavey (2019) points out, even taking into account that this research is about imagined rather than actual behaviour, the fact that so many men are willing to report imagining being able to rape supports feminist arguments that the building blocks of rape exist within or alongside normative heterosexuality rather than being a problem of a deviant few.

Deploying Foucault to Design and Conduct Empirical Research

Through my research, I was interested in taking a different approach to the place of feminism in contemporary work against sexual violence by approaching feminism as a form of knowledge rather than as an identity or form of political activism. This is not in order to diminish the importance of activism or of organisations or indeed individuals adopting an explicitly feminist identity but because it is a useful approach for the purpose of excavating forms of knowledge that are so embedded in a field they have become logical or uncontested explanation. Specifically, the research was informed by a Foucauldian epistemological approach, and I drew on his methodological strategies to design and conduct the empirical work.

> What is worth retaining above all from this approach is its creativity. We should not seek to extract a method … but rather to identify a certain ethos of investigation, a way of asking questions, a focus not upon why things have happened, but how they happened and the difference that that made in relation to what had gone before. Above all, the aim of such studies is critical but not critique … to identify and describe differences and hence to make criticism possible. (Rose, O'Malley, & Valverde, 2009, p. 26)

The strength of adopting Foucault's methodological approach to guide my empirical work lay in his ethos of investigation, a style of questioning and an intellectual creativity that enabled him to make the familiar and taken-for-granted unfamiliar and hence open to question (Rose et al.,

2009). Indeed, Foucault defined his research and role as a researcher in terms akin to an anthropologist—of his own culture. He stated,

> I could define it as an analysis of the cultural facts characterising our culture. I do in fact seek to place myself outside the culture to which we belong, to analyse its formal conditions in order to make a critique of it, not in the sense of reducing its values, but in order to see how it was actually constituted. (Foucault, 1999, p. 91)

It is this investigative ethos I sought to utilise: the capacity to ask questions that open up taken-for-granted ways of doing and seeing.

It is an approach requiring 'critical engagement' with his ideas, rather than passive attempts to apply them (Skehill, 2007, p. 99). While he did not provide a clear-cut set of methodological steps and continually revised his ideas over the course of his career (Castel, 1994; Dean, 1994; Gutting, 2005b; Osborne, 1994; Skehill, 2007), Foucault did, through reflective accounts based on his empirical studies, lay out a series of methodological 'precautions' that he considered important (Foucault, 1972, 1980b, 1998). I based my decisions about how to design and conduct my study on these strategies together with my reading of his (1975) research on institutionalised forms of knowledges and practices in medicine, the French prison system (1977) and mental asylums (1982). These precautions are based on his epistemological approach to knowledge, power and discourse and essentially enable the researcher to operationalise these ideas as methodological tools.

A central focus through Foucault's empirical work is the specificity of the investigation. His studies of sexuality were to have been about 'a specific type of discourse on sex', appearing in specific times and places—for example in relation to practices to control births (1998, p. 97). His research on the professionalisation and institutionalisation of medicine was specifically a study on the institutionalisation of medicine in the French context. For example, the decrees, legislation, reference to conflicts between the universities and government bodies and documents relating to the origins of these institutions all focus on France and the French political, social and economic context (Foucault, 1975). Where there is reference to medical practices and institutions in other European countries discussion is limited to their influence on French medical education, for example.[6]

Similarly, his research on the practice of punishment—from torture to confinement—is principally a study of the birth of the French prison system with careful attention to local institutions and practices—descriptions of prison routines, regulations and timetables for example (Foucault, 1977). In his methodological reflections Foucault referred to this as the methodological strategy or 'precaution' of starting from 'local centers of power–knowledge' (Foucault, 1998, p. 97). This focus on local, rather than centralised, sites enables analysis of the specificity and contingency of the knowledge and discourses produced. Foucault's 'rule' about the polyvalence of discourses, for example, draws attention to the variability within a single discourse, depending on where and how it is deployed, while the 'rule of continual variations' draws attention to the modifications and shifts in knowledge–power relations. The same discourse can have multiple, even opposing, effects, depending on who is speaking and acting and the nature of the institution from which they speak. Importantly, he argued that it is at the extremities—in local centres—that discourse is the most unstable and thus susceptible to change. However, while the focus is local, Foucault makes clear that identification of a discursive formation requires collection and analysis of a range of texts and documents, rather than a single document or document type (Foucault, 1972; Hall, 2004).

Therefore, the research objective was to examine contemporary policy and practices to establish the current position and influence of feminist discourses in the field of sexual assault service provision. Achieving this objective in the contemporary context involved identifying and analysing discourses that intersect with feminist discourses and affect the production of specialist sexual assault services. The research questions formulated to establish this were as follows: (1) What is a sexual assault service? (2) What is a sexual assault worker? (3) What do sexual assault workers do? (4) How have sexual assault services, workers and practice techniques been produced?

[6] However, when it pertains to the corpus of medical knowledge of the late 18th and early 19th—the treatises, nosological charts, the debates over the nature of fevers—the archive broadens considerably. This is not surprising given that, while the specificities of the French political and social context molded medical institutions into a particular shape; the body of knowledge they incorporated was drawn from a European wide rather than specifically French tradition.

Research Design

Provision of sexual assault services are the responsibility of Australia's state and territory governments, rather than the federal government. This means that while there are some similarities that run across Australian services, such as employment of paid rather than volunteer counsellors and long standing receipt of government funding) there are differences particularly given that the other systems that respond to sexual assault such as the legal, police and health systems are also state based. For example, in Victoria all services (whether government or NGO) belong to and adhere to the policies and practices one peak body (Victorian CASA Forum, 2019) whereas in New South Wales (NSW) each have their own peak bodies, meetings, networks and policy guidelines. Similarly, the relative proportion of NGO compared to government services varies. Western Australia for example has one hospital based crisis service in the capital city with the remainder of the state serviced predominantly by NGO's compared to South Australia where most services are government based.[7] These types of differences are reflect historical circumstances and the specific context in which the services developed (Carmody, 1995). For example whether a liberal (conservative) or labour (progressive) state government was in power at the time services developed, the makeup and terms of reference of the various committees set up to examine the issue of sexual violence during the 1970s and 1980s.

Given the aim of my study was to examine institutionalised knowledge production (via service provision) I decided to focus my investigation on one state, which I approached as a local site of power–knowledge. I chose the state of NSW which as Australia's most populous state[8] (almost a third of Australia's population reside here) has the largest network of sexual assault services, with well over 60 services across the state.[9] In comparison Victoria Australia's second most populous state which has 15 services

[7] Yarrow Place, part the South Australian health department is the primary service in that state (SA Health, 2019). Western Australia's Sexual Assault Resource Centre is based in a major public hospital in Perth (WA Government, n.d.), while the NGO responses are provided through a number of different service and funding models (Women's Community Health Network WA, 2020).

[8] The total population of Australia's is 25,364,3000, of which 8,089,5000 live in NSW Statistics (Australian Bureau of Statistics, 2019).

[9] The size of the services does vary though, from large urban services to small services that may employ only two or three counsellors.

(CASA Forum, 2019) and Tasmania a small state with two services only. (Tasmanian Government, n.d.).

The research focused most extensively at the level of service delivery as this enabled examination of practices of power at the extremities where discourses have been institutionalised within local policies and practices. The data selected to form the library of documents reflect this focus and comprise the following: texts produced from interviews conducted with practitioners; publicly available documents produced by the selected services and from within the sector such as brochures, website material, manuals, annual reports and publications; and governance documents such as policy and procedure manuals. These documents and texts vary in focus and intention (see Table 2.1). For example, service brochures are documents whose focus is external in that their message is aimed at potential clients of these services (that is victim of sexual violence), at other service providers who may refer victims to a sexual assault service and, to some extent, at the broader community. While a service brochure

Table 2.1 The library of documents

Category	*Function*	*Types of documents collected*
Programmatic documents	Set out the mechanisms or techniques that give services a particular shape and form	Policy and procedure manuals Job descriptions Annual reports Interagency guidelines Funding documents
Brochures	Target service users (victims), workers from other agencies and the general public	Service brochures Website material, for example, 'About us' pages
Specialist knowledge documents	Documents produced within the field and that target players within the field (that is, practitioners, policy analysts)	Training manuals Research reports Website material from the key training body (NSW Health Education Centre Against Violence)
Practitioner interview texts	Interview questions designed to access types of knowledge practices enacted by practitioners in their day-to-day work Enable access to knowledge/ practices not captured in formal policy documents	Produced from the interview transcripts of 30 interviews with sexual assault practitioners
Key informant interviews	Provided specific information that was missing from policy documents and other written records	Typed summaries of the four interviews

communicates to the public (or sectors of the public), 'This is who we are and what we do', governance documents carefully set out the mechanisms or techniques that build services of a particular shape and form, including the characteristic requirements of the workers. The practitioner interview texts enabled access to applied knowledge and practices that may not be present in formal documents such as policy directives. The combination of documents and individual interviews enabled a more complete picture of how practices are enacted in institutional settings. Key informant interviews were conducted to fill gaps in documentary records. For example, to assist in understanding current as well as changes over time in broader organisational structures (such as the internal organisation of the policy unit that administers NSW Health sexual assault services and changes in name and responsibilities of a key training organisation).

To this end, I conducted 30 onsite semi-structured, in-depth interviews with practitioners recruited from 10 NSW sexual assault services selected to represent the diversity of the sector (urban rural, non-government and government). I designed the interview questions to elicit the types of knowledge practices that practitioners used in their day-to-day work. I asked participants their views on the causes and consequences of sexual violence, about the practice models or approaches they used, the types of work-based training they considered important and their observations about knowledge and practices across the sector, including any changes over time. I positioned these interviews in the research as 'social texts' that produced examples of knowledge practices, rather than as the stories or accounts of the experiences of individuals. I also asked participants a series of questions about their professional background such as their qualifications, training and length of time in their current position and a brief overview of prior employment.

To assist with the production of these texts from the interview transcripts, I used NVivo, a qualitative research software programme, to sort and collate the transcripts into documents that drew together data from across multiple questions on a particular topic or issue. For example, I collated the data into separate documents organised by theme, such as trauma, practice interventions, feminist analysis of sexual violence and so on. I divided each document again according to key concepts, for example, into gendered power and offender responsibility with feminist analyses. The production of these documents was particularly useful in making visible the representation of major discourses or knowledge practices across the texts.

To analyse the documents and interview texts, I used questions adapted from Foucault's (1972) 'rules' for identifying the formation of subjects, objects, concepts and strategies that constitute a discourse. These rules lay out areas of analysis for each of the elements that together comprise a discourse or discursive formation. To illustrate, one of the rules about the production of subjects is that in part they are formed through the institutional sites in which they are located. Another rule, which Foucault (1972) termed 'the grids of specification' (p. 41), is that discursive objects are produced through the ways they are divided, related and derived from each other. Some rules are posed as questions—for example, 'Who can speak?', and others are made up of a series of sub-questions.

The following outlines the specific questions asked of the library of documents, to illuminate 'regimes of truth' and 'practices of power' in the field of sexual assault service provision.

The Subject (Practitioner)

1. What is the character of the sexual assault worker?
2. What institutional sites do they speak from?
3. What 'truth' does the sexual assault worker speak, from where does she derive the authority to do so and how does she know she speaks the truth?
4. What differentiates the sexual assault worker from other groups involved with victims of sexual violence?
5. How have techniques and strategies of power produced the specific character of the sexual assault practitioner?

The Object (Victim)

1. How are victims of different types of sexual assault divided, contrasted, regrouped and derived from each other as objects?
2. Where have these current objects of sexual assault emerged from?

The Concept (Sexual Assault)

1. What assumptions do the documents and texts presuppose when articulating, 'What is sexual violence'?
2. How are discourses from one field transferred to another?
3. What statements, though they belong to other discourses, are active in the discursive field under analysis?

The Strategy (Techniques of Power)

1. What strategies have been deployed to put the discourse to work?
2. What mechanisms (procedures for investigation and research, methods of observation and techniques of registration) have put into circulation the discourse of 'truth' the sexual assault practitioner speaks?

The particular documents and sections of documents analysed depended on the question asked. For example, to establish the 'character' of the sexual assault worker, I focused on the recruitment documents; I selected parts of the programmatic documents and some sections of the interview texts, in particular a document I had produced in NVivo that collated demographic data about practitioners' professional backgrounds and trajectories, and exported them into the field of sexual assault. The question, and related questions, devised to establish the 'truth they speak' focused in more detail on the interview texts.

Historical Development of a Field of Feminist Practice

In this section, I trace the historical development of feminist knowledge practices in the sexual assault services sector from the 1970s to today. I establish the pivotal role accorded second-wave feminism in bringing the issue of sexual violence into the Australian public and political arena and identify feminist political activism as the dominant motif in these accounts. In so doing, I highlight the strategies, mechanisms and knowledge formations that characterise accounts of feminist activism over this period. The aim is to illuminate the production of a field with a particular shape and form and location. The types of historical accounts include those produced by women who worked in, and were part of, the early development of sexual assault services and histories of feminist women's services. The histories of 'femocracies' also contain accounts of the development of the sexual assault field, with a focus on the work of feminist bureaucrats.

Like most other Western countries, sexual assault and rape crisis organisations developed in Australia during the 1970s and 1980s. While some organisations began on a voluntary basis government funding began relatively early in Australia with the Whitlam Government made federal funding, administered through the States, available in 1975 for the establishment of rape crisis centres (Carmody, 1995; Hewitt & Worth, n.d.).[10] The state based nature of the services means there is variation across the country as particular models of service delivery in each state emerged from a combination of local factors and developments in the federal context (Carmody, 1997, p. 453; Hewitt & Worth, n.d.).[11] For example, in some states government task-forces or inquiries were formed to investigate the issue of rape and to guide types of service development, including location (hospitals versus community centres for example) and management. Consequently, while there are some overall similarities, there are also variations in sexual assault policies and service provision.

Histories of feminist activism in the development of a sexual assault services sector typically divide activities into two discrete periods: the first in the 1970s, which focused on adult rape, and the second in the 1980s, which focused on child sexual assault. In NSW, as in most other states and territories, the government response was to set up taskforces to investigate the issues and propose solutions. The first, the NSW Task Force on Care for Victims of Sexual Offences (1978) focused on adult rape, while the second, the NSW Child Sexual Assault Task Force (1987) focused on child sexual assault.[12] During each period, feminist political activism is

[10] Some Rape Crisis Collectives remained unfunded though. These included the Women against Rape Collective that ran in Melbourne, Victoria until 1979 and the Geelong Rape Crisis Collective, also located in Victoria which remined unfunded until 1982 (Hewitt & Worth, n.d.).

[11] In some cases, state responses were prompted by a local situation such as a hospital refusing to treat a rape victim. Examples of other locally based changes and responses include a newly appointed Victorian police surgeon) requesting and receiving permission to examine rape victims in a Melbourne hospital rather than in the police station as had been the case until 1977 Other factors influencing service development include the election of respective state governments and the particular platforms on which they came to power. As an example, the Victorian Labor government came to power in 1982 on a platform of promoting women's issues and consequently established sexual assault services across the state (Hewitt & Worth, n.d.).

[12] Both taskforces produced reports that were used to guide the development of sexual assault services: the first, *Care for Victims of Sexual Offences: Report of the Inter-Departmental Task Force, February 1978* (1978), and the second, *Report of the New South Wales Child*

positioned as instrumental in bringing these issues to the public and community arena in responding to victims and in pressuring governments to act (Breckenridge, 1992, 1999; Carmody, 1995; Sawer, 1990).

The 1970s are depicted as an era of great mobilisation within the women's movement in Australia, an era of campaigns, protests and the mushrooming of) grassroots women's groups. Much has been made of the role of the 'speak-out' as a technique of politicisation in these early years of the women's movement. Indeed, in accounts of women's political activism in NSW, a two-day speak-out held in Sydney as part of International Women's Day 1974 is accorded a central role in the establishment of the first services in NSW for victims of rape and domestic violence. Anne Summers (cited in Carmody, 1995), a key figure in Australian feminism, recounts that after hearing woman after woman speak about their experiences of violence, a group of activist women, including herself, decided they had to do something in response. As a result, Elsie, the first women's refuge, began in an inner Sydney squat, and the Sydney Rape Crisis Collective (SRCC) was established later the same year.

Initially run on a voluntary basis and later with federal and state government financial assistance, the SRCC was the first organised support for victims of sexual assault in NSW (Carmody, 1995; Cooper, n.d).[13] Workers at the centre provided crisis telephone counselling and support, accompanied victims to hospital, police and court, and ran weekly self-defence classes, while at the same time undertaking political campaigns on issues such as rape in marriage, sexual harassment, childhood sexual assault and rape by professionals such as medical practitioners.

Typically, issues reported by victims via the telephone counselling line formed the basis of political campaigns, often in collaboration with other women's organisations (Carmody, 1995). Some campaigns were local, such as the sexual harassment campaign, run with the Women's Officer from a local university after a number of women reported experiencing harassment on campus. Other campaigns had a national focus, such as the campaign about marital rape organised with Rape Crisis collectives across

Sexual Assault Task Force to the Hon. Neville Wran, Q.C., M.P, Premier of New South Wales, March 1985 (1987).

[13] From 1975, the collective received some, though initially quite limited, government funding through a federal grant during the era of the Whitlam Labor government and later through the Women's Health programme grants. There was, however, considerable debate from within the collective about accepting government funding (SRCC, 1994, p. 9). The debate was markedly similar to the concerns raised in the contemporary literature.

Australia (SRCC, 1994, pp. 9–12). By using their accumulated knowledge, the SRCCs were able to apply political pressure on the government by speaking publicly about their knowledge of the poor treatment experienced by victims from police, hospitals and the legal system (Carmody, 1992, 1995).

SRCC was the only sexual assault centre in NSW until the late 1970s, when the NSW Government inquiry into adult rape resulted in sexual assault centres being established in nine public hospitals located in three major metropolitan cities. SRCC had played an instrumental role in the political campaigns that led to this taskforce and had initially joined the working party convened to implement its recommendations but resigned in protest when it became apparent the centres were to be located in hospitals. Rape victims, they protested, were not ill and did not require 'treatment'.

Located in the hospitals' social work departments, these centres were initially limited to providing immediate medical care and crisis counselling to rape victims. At first, they were little more than an after-hours crisis response provided by staff in the respective hospitals' social work departments. Until the latter part of the 1980s, these sexual assault centres,[14] together with SRCC, were the only services in the state. There were no services for victims of sexual assault in rural or regional areas of NSW until the mid-1980s. Often neglected in accounts of service development are the volunteer committees that operated in some rural areas. These were typically set up and run by staff from community health centres, hospitals and women's centres, who volunteered their time to provide support to rape victims such as accompanying them to local police stations and advocating on their behalf (Women's Health Policy Review Committee, 1985, p. 228).

While the feminist movement of the 1970s is represented as a grassroots movement that applied pressure *to* government from *outside*, accounts of the 1980s highlight feminist activism both inside and outside the state. These accounts introduce a new category of feminist, known in Australia as the 'femocrat', who worked from *within* government to

[14]These Centre's were initially—and very briefly referred to as Sexual Offences Referral Centers (SORC's) and then by the 'friendlier term' HELP centres. Adoption of the term sexual assault centre's (SAC's) appears in the early 1980s and coincides with the gradual introduction of dedicated teams of sexual assault workers who operated separately from the generic social work departments (Carmody, 1995).

achieve change. Femocrats worked in senior roles within state and federal government bureaucracies, typically in positions created during the Whitlam era[15] as 'women's issues', and these positions became part of the political and policy agenda. The ensuing policy machinery included women's advisors, women's advisory committees, women's health units and women's coordination units (Franzway, Court, & Connell, 1989; Sawer, 1990). In accounts of the development of the field of sexual assault in NSW, the Sexual Assault Committee appears as the primary strategy used by femocrats to politicise and respond to the issue of child sexual assault (Carmody, 1992, 1995; Franzway et al., 1989; Sawer, 1990). This committee, an evolution of the working party that had been set up in the late 1970s to establish the hospital sexual assault centres, came under the direction of the NSW Government's Women's Coordination Unit. With membership including representatives from the NSW Department of Health sexual assault centres, SRCC and police and legal systems, the committee provided a centralised body through which local services could report on patterns, trends and issues happening 'on the ground' (Carmody, 1995, p. 165).

Equally prominent in histories of 1980s feminism are the mobilising strategies adopted by grassroots feminists working outside government. A powerful new strategy, the 'incest collective', was introduced as an important form of collective mobilisation. Among the most influential of these collectives in NSW was the Women Against Incest Collective (WAIC). According to Burke (1992), one of the original members, the collective formed in 1983 after the women's health centre in South Western Sydney called for a meeting of feminists in community and government agencies in response to the growing number of victims of child sexual assault seeking assistance. The 'collective' is typically associated with—if not emblematic of—grassroots feminist activism. The non-hierarchical, collective structure and decision-making process was a deliberate mechanism for embedding radical feminist politics in organisational practices. As such, it represented a challenge to the way the patriarchal state and associated systems, structures and organisations operated. However, the histories of both the femocrats and grassroots feminist organisations emphasise WAIC

[15] The Whitlam era refers to the period during the 1970s when the federal Labor government under Prime Minister Gough Whitlam introduced wide-reaching social reforms. This included the creation of women's advisory, policy and coordination positions in federal and state governments.

as made up of feminists working in *both* grassroots organisations and in government positions, including workers from the hospital-based sexual assault centres and refuge, rape crisis and women's health centres (e.g. Breckenridge, 1992; Burke, 1992; Carmody, 1995; Cora, 1992; Sawer, 1990). This is an important point because it suggests that feminists working outside and within the state apparatus were, at least in practice if not in an ideological position, not always quite as strictly dichotomised as 'received' histories suggest.[16]

In addition, there appears a subtle shift in the respective roles accorded the incest collective and the earlier speak-outs. Although both involved mobilisation by groups of feminists and shared the non-hierarchical structure emblematic of second-wave grassroots feminism, their overall purpose appears to diverge. Whereas the 'speak-out' was a mechanism for women to speak about their own experiences of violence, the incest collective, or at least WAIC, appears to have been initiated by workers hearing about victims' experiences. The purpose of this collective is described as a way for workers to support each other in their work with incest victims (Burke, 1992), to raise awareness of incest and lobby for counselling and support services (Cora, 1992) and to pressure the state government to form a taskforce (Sawer, 1990). Although some workers may have experienced incest themselves, the purpose of the collective was to support their work with victims, to lobby for services based on the stories they were hearing and to pressure government on behalf of those victims. The reason I highlight this is to suggest that the phenomenon of practitioner—or organisation-led interventions—at the expense of survivor-led activism that informs critiques of professionalisation is not an entirely contemporary 'problem'. While I would not want to overstate the point, the practice of workers from a collective advocating for or speaking on behalf of victims does not seem entirely removed from more contemporary, if more formalised, practices.

There appears to be a degree of overlap in the strategies developed by grassroots feminists and those working within the state to politicise sexual assault and to make demands for public resources. The 'phone-in', for example, was a strategy adopted by feminists across the community/government divide. Typically, this involved using the media of the day to

[16] For examples of different accounts and reflections on the historical conflicts within different strands of Australian feminism during this period, see Breckenridge (1992), Eisenstein (1996), Sawer (1990), Summers (1999) and Weeks (1993).

publicise the chosen issue—in this case incest—including details of a subsequent period when women were asked to phone in about their experiences. Two phone-ins held during 1984 are accorded particular significance in the development of the sexual assault services sector. The NSW Government Sexual Assault Committee orchestrated a phone-in as part of their month-long NSW-wide campaign *No-one Deserves to be Raped*,[17] in which women were asked to phone in, over a three-day period, about gaps in services and with suggestions for reform. The accounts of these activities focus on the lack of services in rural areas for women and children (Carmody, 1995). The other phone-in was organised by WAIC and publicised using the slogan *Break the Silence* (Breckenridge, 1992; Burke, 1992). Also held over a three-day period, this phone-in has been described as not only an important method of collecting information, but as a 'political act in itself', a strategy for educating the community and mobilising feminists (Walby, 1985, cited in Breckenridge, 1992). The accounts of this phone-in focus on the number of women who reported experiences of incestuous abuse in childhood and the lack of support services available to these women.

In a recurring motif, the NSW Government's inquiry into and subsequent *Report of the New South Wales Child Sexual Assault Task Force* (1987) is attributed to one or both of these campaigns (Breckenridge, 1992; Franzway et al., 1989; Sawer, 1990). The outcome of this taskforce was the establishment of sexual assault centres throughout NSW, as well as worker training and policy positions. This included a Sexual Assault Policy Analyst in the Department of Health, whose position encompassed the coordination and development of 22 new government sexual assault centres. Most of these services, particularly in the outer areas of Sydney, were located in community health centres rather than hospitals. Many broadened their employment base beyond social work to include a range of professions, and, unlike the earlier services, all were set up to meet the needs of both child and adult victims. By 1986, the number of Department of Health sexual assault centres had increased from nine to 31, with 19 of the new services in rural areas (Department of Health NSW, 1988, p. 15). By 2005, there were more than 50 NSW Health sexual assault services (NSW Health, 2005).

[17] Part of the campaign involved committee members travelling to rural areas to hold public forums about sexual assault (Carmody, 1995).

Funding was also designated to establish community-based, non-government child sexual assault services, administered through the newly formed NSW Child Protection Council (Breckenridge, 1992; Sawer, 1990). The women's collectives that had formed around the issue of incest, along with other women's organisations, began to apply for this funding. In 1986, women from those organisations who had secured funding formed the Incest Services Network (ISN). In 1995, the ISN, which by then comprised 24 services, became the Child and Adolescent Sexual Abuse Counsellors (CASAC), with services based in Sydney and in regional areas of NSW (CASAC, 2007). In 1998 SRCC became the NSW Rape Crisis Centre (NSWRCC) with service expansion in the 2000s including the introduction of online as well as telephone crisis counselling, expanded training programmes, research and a face-to-face community based counselling service (NSWRCC, 2008; R&DVSA, 2019c).

In addition to the actual services, an important part of the establishment of the field of sexual assault was the introduction of worker training, a new policy agency and legislative reforms. In 1985, sexual assault training positions were established in the Department of Family and Community Services (the state statutory child protection body), in the Department of Education and in both government- and community-based sexual assault centres. In addition to overseeing the funding of the community-based child sexual assault centres, NSW Child Protection Council[18] was responsible for monitoring legal reforms (including the new mandatory notification of child sexual abuse reform) and for providing worker training and community education (Breckenridge, 1992; Sawer, 1990). By 1988, the Sexual Assault Education Unit had developed from the initial two government (NSW Health) training positions (Carmody, 1995). Reflecting an evolving role, the unit was renamed the Women's Health and Sexual Assault Unit in 1990, and now, as the Education Centre Against Violence (ECAV), has a number of training portfolios including domestic violence, Aboriginal family violence, child protection and cultural equity, in addition to sexual assault (ECAV, n.d.).

[18] The NSW Child Protection Council operated from 1985 until 1995 when it was replaced by the NSW Commission for Children and Young People and in 2015 by the Office of the Advocate for Children and Young People. The role in advocating for and ensuring the safety and well-being of children and young people has remained broadly similar across these organisations.

Tracing the Architecture of Contemporary NSW Sexual Assault Services

From a single organisation in 1974, the NSW sexual assault services sector now encompasses a complex assemblage of overlapping and hierarchically organised bodies typical of contemporary social service provision in welfare states. This includes training bodies such as the ECAV, policy and management infrastructure embedded in NSW Health, peak bodies such as CASAC Inc.[19] and a number of committees and organisational bodies set up to facilitate work between sexual assault services and other key institutions that respond to sexual violence. The latter include police, legal and medical practitioners, and statutory child protection services (Office of the Director of Public Prosecutions, 2015). Under this umbrella are more than 50 NSW Health sexual assault services[20] located in urban and rural areas throughout the state (NSW Health, 2018), a network of non-government child sexual assault services (CASAC Inc, 2016) and Rape and Domestic Violence Services Australia (R&DVSA), a large NGO that now incorporates NSW Rape Crisis.[21] The introduction of Child Protection

[19] CASAC Inc. represents the community-based child sexual assault counselling and support services. Some CASAC services such as Rosebank and The West St Centre are 'stand alone' sexual assault services while others (sometimes a sole worker service) form part of larger NGO's which provide a number of different types of services.

[20] NSW Health is the current name for the former Department of Health NSW. Likewise, the term 'sexual assault service has replaced 'sexual assault centre'.

[21] In 2013, the name of NSWRCC changed to Rape and Domestic Violence Services Australia (R&DVSA). The name change was made to reflect the organisation's increasing national focus and expanded range of services (R&DVSA, 2019c). This included the service receiving federal government funding to provide a national sexual assault and domestic violence telephone support line (1800 Respect) and to provide national telephone support and counselling to survivors of child sexual abuse in institutions. While NSW Rape Crisis continues to exist, it is now one of a number of services provided by R&DVSA. In the ever-changing funding climate, R&DVSA lost funding for the 1800 Respect line in late 2017. The funding for survivors of child sexual abuse was made available to selected sexual assault services, across Australia, including R&DVSA, as part of the Royal Commission into Institutional Responses to Child Sexual Abuse (2017) which ran for five years from 2013. While the Royal Commission attracted intense media and public attention and has done much to bring the issue of sexual abuse by clergy into public consciousness. I would make the point though that sexual assault services had been working with survivors of institutional child abuse for many years prior to this as well as working to have the issue brought to public attention. The more recent funding has assisted often already thinly stretched services to cope with the increased numbers of survivors seeking assistance as a result of the Commission rather than substantially changing the nature or type interventions or assistance provided by these services.

Units (CPUs) into the NSW field is a relatively recent change, dating back to the mid- to late-1990s. In contrast to child sexual assault services, CPUs were set up to respond to all forms of child abuse, physical and emotional abuse and neglect, as well as child sexual abuse. They are located in four major teaching hospitals[22] in the same geographical areas as the adult hospital-based sexual assault services and provide a service to child victims in these areas. Collectively, these services provide a range of responses to sexual violence, including 24-hour crisis response, counselling, advocacy and group work, medical assistance and community education work (CASAC Inc, 2007, 2016; NSW Health, 2018; Rosebank, 2019; R&DVSA, 2019b). See Fig. 2.1 for a diagrammatic representation of the current NSW sexual assault services sector.[23]

The administration, coordination and development of the NSW Health sexual assault services are currently managed through the NSW Health Prevention and Response to Violence, Abuse and Neglect (PARVAN) unit, facilitated through regular statewide meetings in which all services have representation. PARVAN as the name suggests develops NSW Health policy and responses designed to identify, prevent and respond to the issues of violence, abuse and neglect including child and adult sexual assault, domestic violence, Aboriginal family violence and the physical, emotional abuse and neglect of children medical and forensic examinations in relation to sexual assault, domestic violence and child abuse, (NSW Health, 2019, 2020a). NSW Rape Crisis continues to provide a 24 hour telephone and online counselling response to anyone affected by sexual assault in NSW, as part of the range of services and programmes now provided by Rape and Domestic Violence Services Australia; the later including community based face to face counselling in a number of NSW women's health services and extensive community and work place training programmes (R&DVSA, 2019a).

[22] Three are in the major NSW children's hospitals, and the fourth is in a general hospital.

[23] This figure has been designed to capture only key features of the sector in a visual format. It does not for example include specific local, state or national committees that individual services may have representation on as part of their advocacy work. For example, Rape and Domestic Violence Services Australia (R&DVSA) has representation on state as well as national peak bodies; the latter includes the National Association of Services Against Sexual Violence a national peak body to which some state based services belong (NASASV, n.d.; Women's Health NSW, 2020).

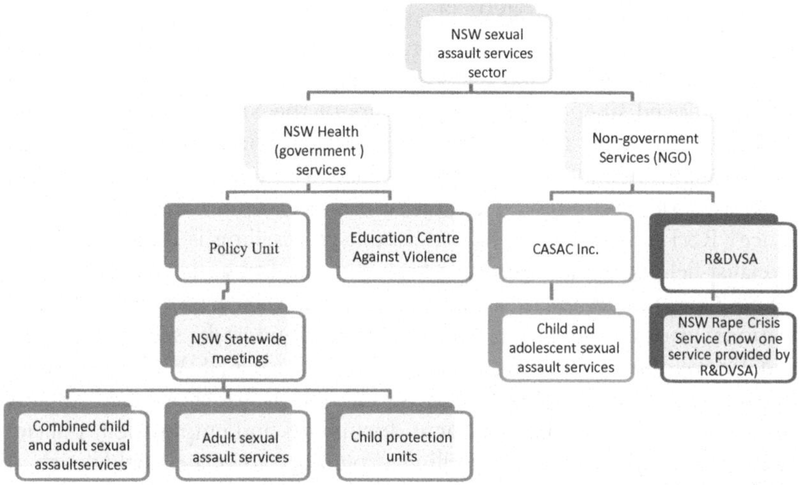

Fig. 2.1 The contemporary NSW field of sexual assault service provision. (Source: Egan, 2019)

All services are funded by the government and, consequently, are subject to the types of regulations associated with 'publicness' in the Australian context, including funding reviews, monitoring of outcomes and specified criteria for service. Non-government (NGO) sexual assault services are not typically positioned as 'public' services. However, in the Australian context these services are typically funded by and therefore subject to regulation through the state. Most CASAC services for example receive core funding through schemes administered by the NSW Department of Communities and Justice whose responsibilities include the assessment and investigation of reports of child abuse and the care and protection of abused children (NSW Communities & Justice, 2020). Similarly, NSW Rape Crisis is funded by NSW Health (R&DVSA, 2019d) as are the women's health services in which some CASAC services are located.[24] There are no private or for-profit sexual assault services.

[24]NGO's often receive funding from a number of different sources, including one off grants, funding from different government departments philanthropic donations. In addition reoccurring funding may come from more than one government department (for example state and/or federal government departments), depending on the specific programmes provided by the NGO.

Sexual assault work in NSW, like other Australian states and territories, is a highly professionalised area of practice. Unlike some rape crisis centres in the United Kingdom and United States, volunteer counsellors have not been employed since the very early years of the SRCC. Indeed, student placements at Rape and Domestic Violence Services Australia are open only to applicants undertaking postgraduate (for example Masters level in social work or psychology) with at least three years prior counselling experience (R&DVSA, 2019e). Sexual assault counselling is understood as a specialist field of work requiring a high degree of training. Workers across the NGO and government sectors are required to have tertiary level qualifications, prior counselling experience, and to undertake specialist professional development training on an ongoing basis (NSW Health, 2005, 2020b; R&DVSA, 2019b). Sexual assault work is not considered suitable for new graduates, with recruitment documents and employment policies typically specifying prior counselling experience in related fields such as child protection, domestic violence or women's health. These types of specifications are consistent with the career trajectories of the workers I interviewed, the majority of whom were from social work or psychology backgrounds with a significant number holding postgraduate qualifications, usually in counselling-related areas, such as a master's degree in counselling, with their trajectories into sexual assault counselling often coming via work in related fields such of domestic violence, child protection and women's health services.

Through analysis of the service and sector documents and the practitioner interviews, I found feminist knowledge of sexual violence to hold an authoritative, almost naturalised, position in the contemporary NSW field of sexual assault service provision. This was to the extent that the definition of sexual assault, used in a key government policy document governing service provision, was not only based on a feminist analysis of sexual assault but presented as a factual account of 'what sexual assault is' rather than as a theory or perspective. As I lay out in the next chapter, these ideas about 'what sexual assault is' enable the basic rules of engagement or policies that underpin sexual assault service provision. Feminist ideas are evident, for example, in policies stipulating that sexual assault services work only with victims and not with offenders, in the premise that responsibility lies with the offender and not the victim, and in the statements (evident in policies, procedure manuals, fact sheets and other information sources) that sexual assault is a crime of violence.

Analysis of the practitioner interview texts enabled me to build a more nuanced picture of how feminism operates in the day-to-day work of sexual assault practitioners in the field. The concepts of male power, violence, structural gender inequality and locating responsibility with the abuser were replicated across the texts as the core concepts practitioners used to articulate what sexual assault is and why it happens. Deployed through the technique of counselling, these key feminist concepts produce a distinctive type of practice: first, practices that work with the concept of power and focus on enabling the victim to regain the power lost through the experience of sexual assault; second, practices that work with the self-blame often experienced by victims; and third, practices that work between the individual and the structures and systems that support sexual assault. Each of these techniques requires practitioners to work with the effects that sexual assault has on individual victims through deployment of a structural conceptual lens of sexual assault. In this way, the practice of counselling is not necessarily indicative of feminist decline but operates in this field as a component of the feminist political project.

Running parallel to this structural feminist understanding, sexual assault as trauma emerged as a dominant and again naturalised concept in the work of sexual assault practitioners in this field. The concept of psychological trauma codified in the diagnoses of PTSD and complex trauma—that is, knowledge associated with psychiatry and medical science—did appear initially to be a contradictory presence in a field of practice with origins in second-wave feminist politics and that had campaigned *against* the treatment of women by professions such as psychiatry. I found that it was practitioners' understanding of sexual assault as an ontological assault, as a violation of the self, that helped make sense of the frequent recourse to 'trauma'. Sexuality as central to one's identity is, as Foucault has shown us, a deeply held cultural belief in contemporary Western society. Likewise, a psychological understanding of the self as an interiorised entity of motivations, desires and beliefs underlies much popular, professional and academic discourse (Rose, 1996). Predicated on such an understanding of personhood, the concept of psychological trauma was deployed through the interview texts to express this profound violation of the self and to make visible the seriousness and harm of sexual assault.

However, I found the uptake of trauma as feminist practice simultaneously enabling and problematic. The deployment of 'complex trauma', for example, was used by practitioners as a strategy to disrupt the pathologisation experienced by adults who had experienced sexual assault during their childhoods, especially through contact with mental health systems. As such, this can be and was understood by practitioners as a longstanding technique of feminist political practice that aims to ensure sexual assault victims are believed, not blamed, and treated with respect. Yet as I illustrate in Chapter 4, the particular category of victim, the 'adult survivor' produced through complex trauma, is a problematic category. The unproblematic framing of problems 'adult survivors' experience in adulthood as symptoms of 'untreated childhood trauma' holds the potential for producing a quite constrained subject position, one in which the 'adult survivor' is afforded little agency: She becomes a 'vulnerable' individual whose early experiences of abuse leave them perpetually at 'risk' of further harm. To help 'make sense' of this finding, I drew on the small but robust body of post-structural feminist research that critically engages with the normative ideas about psychologised harm and trauma that inform most contemporary feminist understandings of adults sexually abused as children. Particularly useful is the research that unpacks the normative ideas about (hetero) sexuality and child development that underpin the 'adult survivor'. This analysis highlights the extent to which the attribution of current problems, particularly relationship problems, to childhood sexual abuse is based on assumptions about 'normal' women and the 'normal' developmental pathway to healthy adult sexuality. To argue that it is a lack of theorisation of normative (hetero) sexuality has enabled, at least in part, the constrained subject positions available to the 'adult survivor' present in my research.

Further, I conclude that theorisation of trauma as having co-opted contemporary feminist knowledge/s of sexual violence does not adequately explain the normative place of trauma or how it operates in the local field. Trauma was represented consistently in the interview texts as compatible with feminist practices. Taking this representation as a departure point, I analysed the textual evidence produced through my empirical work and, utilising Foucault's methodological strategy of the polyvalence of discourse, began from the position that there *was* a level of compatibility between feminism and trauma. From this position, the analytic focus became about *how* feminism and trauma worked together and about how practitioners had integrated trauma and feminist knowledge/practices.

From this analytic position, I was able to make visible the level of agency with which practitioners engaged with trauma. It is an active and knowing engagement rather than a passive acceptance or co-option. There is an awareness demonstrated in the interview texts of how sexual assault as trauma has changed practices and of the potential within-trauma discourse to deprive victims of agency. I argue that this knowingness enables practitioners to interrupt the totalising potential that trauma, like any discourse, possesses.

Through examining the interview texts for representations of interventions with clients and concrete examples of practice models, I identified the neurobiological aspects of trauma knowledge as most actively employed by sexual assault workers. It was their understanding of how trauma affects victims' bodies and minds that practitioners identified as the aspects of trauma and which they deployed as part of their established feminist practice of enabling clients to regain their power and control. Using Foucault's concept of concomitance, I argue that practitioners are able to integrate trauma and feminism because, while they may appear and are often presented as oppositional forms of knowledge, they are based on shared or compatible underlying concepts of embodied subjectivity and a psychologised understanding of the self.

Conclusion

In this chapter, I introduced the concept of approaching feminism as a form of social and discursive knowledge and illustrated the ways this informed both my empirical work and the type of intervention I am seeking to make in relation to how the terms of the debate have been constructed in the academic scholarship. Over the course of the following chapters, I return to and expand on the key research findings introduced here.

References

Attorney General's Department. New South Wales. (2006). *Criminal justice sexual offences taskforce. Responding to sexual assault: The way forward.* Sydney, Australia: Author.

Australian Bureau of Statistics. (2019). *Australian demographic statistics.* Canberra, Australia: Author. Retrieved from www.abs.gov.au/ausstats/abs@.nsf/0/D56C4A3E41586764CA2581A70015893E?Opendocument

Bartky, S. (1988). Foucault, femininity and the modernisation of patriarchal power. In G. Diamond & L. Quinby (Eds.), *Feminism and Foucault. Reflections on resistance* (pp. 61–68). Boston, MA: North Eastern University Press.

Bell, V. (1993). *Interrogating incest: Feminism, Foucault and the law*. London, UK: Routledge.

Beres, M. A., Crow, B., & Gotell, L. (2009). The perils of institutionalization in neoliberal times: Results of a national survey of Canadian sexual assault and rape crisis centres. *Canadian Journal of Sociology, 34*(1), 135–163.

Blagg, H., Bluett-Boyd, N., & Williams, E. (2015). *Innovative models in addressing violence against Indigenous women: State of knowledge paper (ANROWS Landscapes, 08/2015)*. Retrieved from http://www.anrows.org.au/publication/innovative-models-in-addressing-violence-against-indigenous-women-state-of-knowledge-paper/

Bluett-Boyd, N. (2014). *Victim/survivor-focused justice responses and reforms to criminal court practice: Implementation, current practice and future directions, research report no. 27*. Melbourne, Australia: Australian Institute of Family Studies.

Blyth, J., & Vernan, C. (1992). Victim to survivor: Counselling for recovery to rape. In J. Breckenridge & M. Carmody (Eds.), *Crimes of violence. Australian responses to rape and child sexual assault* (pp. 130–138). North Sydney, Australia: Allen & Unwin.

Bordo, S. (1988). Anorexia nervosa: Psychopathology as the crystallisation of culture. In G. Diamond & L. Quinby (Eds.), *Feminism and Foucault: Reflections on resistance* (pp. 87–117). Boston, MA: North Eastern University Press.

Bordo, S. (1993). Feminism, Foucault and the politics of the body. In C. Ramazanoglu (Ed.), *Up against Foucault* (pp. 179–202). Routledge.

Breckenridge, J. (1992). An exotic phenomenon? Incest and child rape. In J. Breckenridge & M. Carmody (Eds.), *Crimes of violence: Australian responses to rape and child sexual assault* (pp. 18–37). Sydney, Australia: Allen & Unwin.

Breckenridge, J. (1999). Subjugation and silences: The role of the professions in silencing victims of sexual and domestic violence. In J. Breckenridge & L. Laing (Eds.), *Challenging silence: Innovative responses to sexual and domestic violence* (pp. 6–32). St Leonards, Australia: Allen & Unwin.

Breckenridge, J., & Carmody, M. (1992). *Crimes of violence: Australian responses to rape and child sexual assault*. North Sydney, Australia: Allen & Unwin.

Breckenridge, J., & Laing, L. (Eds.). (1999). *Challenging silence. Innovative responses to sexual and domestic violence*. St Leonards, NSW, Australia: Allen & Unwin.

Breckenridge, J., Rees, S., Valentine, K., & Murray, S. (2016). *Meta-evaluation of existing interagency partnerships, collaboration, coordination and/or integrated interventions and service responses to violence against women: Final report*

ANROWS Horizons, 04/2016. Retrieved from www.anrows.org.au/publication/meta-evaluation-of-existing-interagency-partnerships-collaboration-coordination-and-or-integrated-interventions-and-service-responses-to-violence-against-women-final-report/

Brown, W. (2003). Women's studies unbound: Revolution, mourning, politics. *Parrallax, 9*(2), 3–16.

Bumiller, K. (2008). *In an abusive state: How neoliberalism appropriated the feminist movement against sexual violence*. Durham, NJ: Duke University Press.

Burke, C. (1992). Expert on her own story: Working with women's experiences of incest. In J. Breckenridge & M. Carmody (Eds.), *Crimes of violence: Australian responses to rape and child sexual assault* (pp. 109–120). North Sydney, Australia: Allen & Unwin.

Burstow, B. (2005). A critique of posttraumatic stress disorder and the DSM. *Journal of Humanistic Psychology, 45*(4), 429–445.

Burt, M. R. (1980). *Cultural myths and supports for rape*. Journal of Personality & Social Psychology, 38(2), 217–230.

Butler, J. (1990). *Gender trouble: Feminism and the subversion of identity*. New York, NY: Routledge.

Butler, J. (1993). *Bodies that matter: On the discursive limits of 'sex'*. New York, NY: Routledge.

Butler, S. (1985). *Conspiracy of silence: The trauma of incest*. Volcano, CA: Volcano Press.

Campbell, R., Baker, C. K., & Mazurek, T. L. (1998). Remaining radical? Organizational predictors of rape crisis centers' social change initiatives. *American Journal of Community Psychology, 26*(3), 457.

Carmody, M. (1992). Uniting all women: A historical look at attitudes to rape. In J. Breckenridge & M. Carmody (Eds.), *Crimes of violence: Australian responses to rape and child sexual assault* (pp. 18–37). Sydney, Australia: Allen & Unwin.

Carmody, M. (1995). *Site of struggle: The development of sexual assault services in New South Wales, Australia* (Unpublished doctoral dissertation). University of New South Wales, Australia.

Carmody, M. (1997). Submerged voices: Coordinators of sexual assault services speak of their experiences. *Affilia Journal of Women and Social Work, 12*(4), 452–471.

Carmody, M., Evans, S., Krogh, C., Flood, M., Heenan, M., & Ovenden, G. (2009). *Framing best practice: National standards for the primary prevention of sexual assault through education, national sexual assault prevention education project for NASASV*. Sydney, Australia: University of Western Sydney & NASASV.

CASA Forum. (2019). What are the Victorian CASAs? Retrieved from https://www.casa.org.au/about-us/what-are-the-victorian-casas/

Case, J. (1992). Meeting others. Groupwork for children who have been sexually abused. In J. Breckenridge & M. Carmody (Eds.), *Crimes of violence. Australian responses to rape and child sexual assault* (pp. 144–150). North Sydney, Australia: Allen & Unwin.

Castel, R. (1994). 'Problematization' as a mode of reading history. In J. Goldstein (Ed.), *Foucault and the writing of history* (pp. 237–252). Oxford, UK: Blackwell.

Child and Adolescent Sexual Assault Counsellors Inc. (CASAC Inc.). (2007). *Policy and procedure manual.* Sydney, Australia: Author.

Child and Adolescent Sexual Assault Counsellors Inc. (CASAC Inc.). (2016). Submission to the Parliament of NSW Child Protection Inquiry. July 2016. Retrieved from www.parliament.nsw.gov.au/lcdocs/submissions/56171/0104%20CASAC%20Inc%20NSW.pdf

Cooper, N. (n.d.). History—The Sydney women's liberation movement 1970–1975. Retrieved from http://whnsw.asn.au/wp-content/uploads/2016/01/The_Sydney_Womens_Liberation_Movement_1970-1975

Cora, D. (1992). Breaking the silence: Support groups for adult incest survivors. In J. Breckenridge & M. Carmody (Eds.), *Crimes of violence: Australian responses to rape and child sexual assault* (pp. 151–161). North Sydney, Australia: Allen & Unwin.

Corrigan, R. (2014). Why feminist theory matters for feminist practice: The case of rape response. *Politics & Gender, 10*(12), 280–284.

Cox, D. (2008). *Working with Indigenous survivors of sexual assault. ACSSA Wrap, 4.* Melbourne, Australia: Australian Centre for the Study of Sexual Assault, Australian Institute of Family Studies.

Crome, S. (2006). *Male survivors of sexual assault and rape. ACSSA Wrap, 2.* Melbourne, Australia: Australian Centre for the Study of Sexual Assault, Australian Institute of Family Studies.

Cvetkovich, A. (2003). Witnessing things: A response to Sue Grand. *Studies in Gender and Sexuality, 4*(4), 353–362. https://doi.org/10.1080/15240650409349233

Davidson, J., & McNamara, L. (1999). Systems that silence: Lifting the lid on psychiatric institutional sexual abuse. In J. Breckenridge & L. Laing (Eds.), *Challenging silence: Innovative responses to sexual and domestic violence* (pp. 86–102). St Leonards, Australia: Allen & Unwin.

Dean, C., Hardiman, A., & Draper, G. (1998). *National standards of practice manual for services against sexual violence.* Melbourne, Australia: National Association of Services against Sexual Violence Project Team, CASA House.

Dean, M. (1994). *Critical and effective histories. Foucault's methods and historical sociology.* London, UK: Routledge.

Department of Health NSW. (1988). *Sexual assault services: Policy and procedure manual.* Sydney, Australia: Author.

Deveaux, M. (1994). Feminism and empowerment. A critical reading of Foucault. *Feminist Studies, 20*(2), 223–246.

Doyle, S., & Barbato, C. (1999). Justice delayed is justice denied: The experience of women in court as victims of sexual assault. In J. Breckenridge & L. Laing (Eds.), *Challenging silence: Innovative responses to sexual and domestic violence* (pp. 47–58). St Leonards, Australia: Allen & Unwin.

Education Centre Against Violence (ECAV). (n.d.). *Home.* Retrieved from http://www.ecav.health.nsw.gov.au/#

Egan, S. (2019). Excavating feminist knowledges and practices in the field of sexual assault service provision: An Australian case study. *Women's Studies International Forum, 74*(May–June), 169–178. Elsevier. https://doi.org/10.1016/j.wsif.2019.04.001

Eisenstein, H. (1996). *Inside agitators. Australian femocrats and the state.* St Leonards, Australia: Allen & Unwin.

Fergus, L. (2005). Trafficking in women for sexual exploitation. *ACSSA Briefing Paper, 1.* Melbourne, Australia: Australian Centre for the Study of Sexual Assault, Australian Institute of Family Studies.

Fergus, L., & Keel, M. (2005). *Adult victim/survivors of childhood sexual assault, ACSSA Wrap No. 1.* Melbourne, Australia: Australian Centre for the Study of Sexual Assault, Australian Institute of Family Studies.

Foucault, M. (1972). *The archaeology of knowledge & the discourse on language* (A. Sheridan, Trans.). New York, NY: Pantheon Books.

Foucault, M. (1975). *The birth of the clinic: An archaeology of medical perception* (A. S. Smith, Trans.). New York, NY: Vintage.

Foucault, M. (1977). *Discipline and punish: The birth of the prison* (A. Sheridan, Trans.). London, UK: Penguin Books.

Foucault, M. (1980a). Two lectures. In C. Gordon (Ed.), *Power/knowledge: Selected interviews and other writings 1972–1977* (pp. 78–108). New York, NY: Pantheon.

Foucault, M. (1980b). Truth and power. In C. Gordon (Ed.), *Power/knowledge: Selected interviews and other writings 1972–1977* (pp. 109–133). New York, NY: Pantheon.

Foucault, M. (1982). *Madness and civilization: A history of insanity in the age of reason* (R. Howard, Trans.). London, UK: Tavistock.

Foucault, M. (1998). *The will to knowledge: The history of sexuality: 1* (A. Sheridan, Trans.). London, UK: Penguin Books.

Foucault, M. (1999). *Religion and Culture/by Michel Foucault.* Selected and edited by J. R. Carrette. Manchester, England: Manchester University Press.

Foucault, M. (2001). *Fearless speech* (J. Pearson, Trans.). Los Angeles, CA: Semiotext(e).

Franzway, S., Court, D., & Connell, R. W. (1989). *Staking a claim: Feminism, bureaucracy and the state.* North Sydney, Australia: Allen & Unwin.

Fraser, N. (1989). *Unruly practices. Power, discourse and gender in contemporary social theory.* Cambridge, UK: Polity Press.

Frawley, P., Dyson, S., Robinson, S., & Dixon, J. (2015). *What does it take? Developing informed and effective tertiary responses to violence and abuse of women and girls with disabilities in Australia: State of knowledge paper (ANROWS Landscapes, 03/2015).* Retrieved from https://www.anrows.org.au/publication/what-does-it-take-developing-informed-and-effective-tertiary-responses-to-violence-and-abuse-of-women-and-girls-with-disabilities-in-australia-state-of-knowledge-paper/

Freedman, R., & Want, C. (1992). The power of therapy: Working with children who have been sexually abused. In *Crimes of violence. Australian responses to rape and child sexual assault* (pp. 121–129). North Sydney, Australia: Allen & Unwin.

Gavey, N. (2019). *Just sex?: The cultural scaffolding of rape* (2nd ed.). Abingdon, UK and New York, NY: Routledge.

Genovese, A. (2000). The politics of naming: 70s feminisms, genealogy and 'domestic violence'. In R. Walker, K. Brass, & J. Byron (Eds.), *Anatomies of violence: An interdisciplinary investigation* (pp. 115–129). University of Sydney, Australia: The Research Institute of Humanities and Social Sciences.

Gutting, G. (2005a). *Foucault. A very short introduction.* Oxford, UK: Oxford University Press.

Gutting, G. (2005b). Michel Foucault: A user's manual. In G. Gutting (Ed.), *The Cambridge companion to Foucault* (pp. 1–28). Cambridge, UK: Cambridge University Press.

Hall, S. (2004). Foucault and discourse. In C. Seale (Ed.), *Social research methods reader* (pp. 345–349). London, UK: Routledge.

Heenan, M. (2004). *Just "keeping the peace": A reluctance to respond to male partner sexual violence. ACSSA Issues Paper, 1.* Melbourne, Australia: Australian Centre for the Study of Sexual Assault, Australian Institute of Family Studies.

Hemmings, C. (2005). Telling feminist stories. *Feminist Theory, 6*(2), 115–139.

Herman, J. (1981). Father–daughter incest. *Professional Psychology, Research and Practice, 12*(1), 76–80. https://doi.org/10.1037/0735-7028.12.1.76

Hewitt, L., & Worth, C. (n.d.). *Victims like us: The development of the Victorian Centres Against Sexual Assault.* Retrieved from https://www.casa.org.au/about-us/victims-like-us-the-development-of-the-victorian-casas/

Irwin, J., & Thorpe, R. (1996). Women, violence and social change. In J. Irwin & R. Thorpe (Eds.), *Women & violence: Working for change* (pp. 1–15). Sydney, Australia: Hale & Iremonger.

Jones, H., & Cook, K. (2008). *Rape crisis. Responding to sexual violence.* Dorset, UK: Russell House Publishing.

Keel, M., Fergus, L., & Heenan, M. (2005). *Home truths: A conference in review.* Melbourne, Australia: Australian Centre for the Study of Sexual Assault, Australian Institute of Family Studies.

Laing, L. (1992). Other ways of understanding. Training sexual assault workers In J. Breckenridge & M. Carmody (Eds.), *Crimes of Violence. Australian responses to rape and child sexual assault* (pp. 74–85). North Sydney, Australia: Allen & Unwin.

Lamb, S. (1999). Constructing the victim: Popular images and lasting labels. In S. Lamb (Ed.), *New versions of victims: Feminists struggle with the concept* (pp. 108–138). New York, NY and London, UK: New York University Press.

Lay, Y. (2006). Identifying the woman, the client and the victim. *ACSSA Aware, 12*, 15–20. Melbourne, Australia: Australian Centre for the Study of Sexual Assault, Australian Institute of Family Studies.

Leviore, D. (2005). No longer silent. A Study of women's help-seeking decisions and service responses to sexual assault. Canberra, Australia: Australian Institute of Criminology & Office for Women, Australian Government.

Maier, S. L. (2008). Are rape crisis centers feminist organizations? *Feminist Criminology, 3*(2), 82–100. https://doi.org/10.1177/1557085107310623

Mardorossian, C. M. (2002). Towards a new feminist theory of rape. *Signs, 27*(3), 743–775.

Marecek, J. (1999). Trauma talk in feminist clinical practice. In S. Lamb (Ed.), *New versions of victims: Feminist struggle with the concept* (pp. 158–182). New York, NY: New York University Press.

Members of the North Shore Women's Group with, Carmody, M., & Blyth, J. (1992). Your soul on the floor: A Women's rape support group. In J. Breckenridge & M. Carmody (Eds.), *Crimes of violence. Australian responses to rape and child sexual assault* (pp. 162–168). North Sydney, Australia: Allen & Unwin.

Mitra-Kahn, T., Newbigin, C., & Hardefeldt, S. (2016). *Invisible women, invisible violence: Understanding and improving data on the experiences of domestic and family violence and sexual assault for diverse groups of women.* State of knowledge paper (ANROWS Landscapes, DD01/2016. Retrieved from http://www.anrows.org.au/publication/invisible-women-invisible-violence-understanding-and-improving-data-on-the-experiences-of-domestic-and-family-violence-and-sexual-assault-for-diverse-groups-of-women-state-of-knowledge-paper/

Murray, S., & Powell, A. (2008). *Sexual assault and adults with a disability. Enabling recognition, disclosure and a just response.* Melbourne, Australia: Australian Centre for the Study of Sexual Assault, Australian Institute of Family Studies.

NASASV. (n.d.). Home. Retrieved from www.nasasv.org.au/index.htm
National Association of Services Against Sexual Violence. (2000). *National data collection project. Report on the snapshot data collection by Australian services against sexual violence. May–June 2000.* Melbourne, Australia: Author.
Neame, A., & Heenan, M. (2004). *Responding to sexual assault in rural communities.* Melbourne, Australia: Australian Centre for the Study of Sexual Assault, Australian Institute of Family Studies.
NSW Child Sexual Assault Task Force. (1987). *Report of the New South Wales Child Sexual Assault Task Force to the Hon. Neville Wran, Q.C., M.P, Premier of New South Wales, March 1985.* Sydney, Australia: New South Wales Government.
NSW Communities & Justice. (2020). Department of Communities and Justice Strategic Direction 2020–2024, Sydney, Australia: New South Wales Government.
NSW Health. (2005). *Sexual assault services policy and procedure manual (adult).* Sydney, Australia: NSW Health.
NSW Health. (2018). Sexual Assault Services. Retrieved from https://www.health.nsw.gov.au/parvan/sexualassault/Pages/default.aspx
NSW Health. (2019). Integrated prevention and response to violence, abuse and neglect. NSW Health Violence, Abuse and Neglect Redesign Program August 2019 Framework, NSW Ministry of Health St Leonard's, Australia. Retrieved from www.health.nsw.gov.au/parvan/Publications/iparvan-framework.pdf
NSW Health. (2020a). Prevention and response to violence, abuse and neglect. Retrieved from www.health.nsw.gov.au/parvan/Pages/default.aspx
NSW Health. (2020b). *Responding to sexual assault (adult and child) policy and procedures.* Sydney, Australia: NSW Health.
NSW Rape Crisis Centre (NSWRCC). (2008). *Annual report 2007/2008.* Sydney, Australia: Author.
NSW Task Force on Care for Victims of Sexual Offences: New South Wales. Premier's Department. (1978). *Care for victims of sexual offences. Report of the inter-departmental task force, february 1978.* Sydney Australia: Premier's Department.
NSW Violence Against Women Specialist Unit. (2006). *Improving service and criminal justice responses to victims of sexual assault: A report of a state-based consultation with adult victims of sexual assault, services and agencies.* Sydney, Australia: Author.
O'Dell, L. (2003). The 'harm' story in childhood sexual abuse: Contested understandings, disputed knowledges. In P. Reavey & S. Warner (Eds.), *New feminist stories of child sexual abuse: Sexual scripts and dangerous dialogues* (pp. 131–147). London, UK: Routledge.

Office of the Director of Public Prosecutions. (2015). *Annual Report 2014–2015.* Retrieved from https://www.odpp.nsw.gov.au/sites/default/files/attachments/2014-2015-annual-report.pdf

Olle, L. (2005). *Mapping health sector and interagency protocols on sexual assault.* Melbourne, Australia: Australian Centre for the Study of Sexual Assault, Australian Institute of Family Studies.

Osborne, T. (1994). Sociology, liberalism and the historicity of conduct. *Economy and Society, 23*(4), 484–373.

Phillips, R. (2006). Undoing an activist response: Feminism and the Australian government's response to domestic violence. *Critical Social Policy, 26*, 192–219.

Probyn, E. (1998). Re: Generation. Women's studies and the disciplining of ressentiment. *Australian Feminist Studies, 13*(27), 129–136.

Quadara, A., Stathopoulos, M., & Jenkinson, R. (2015). *Establishing the connection [between alcohol and other drug use and sexual victimisation]: State of knowledge paper (ANROWS Landscapes, 06/2015.* Retrieved from https://www.anrows.org.au/publication/establishing-the-connection-between-alcohol-and-other-drug-use-and-sexual-victimisation-state-of-knowledge-paper/

Rape & Domestic Violence Services Australia (R&DVSA). (2019a). 2018/2019 Annual report. Retrieved from www.rape-dvservices.org.au/about/our-governance

Rape & Domestic Violence Services Australia (R&DVSA). (2019b). Our counselling services. Retrieved from www.rape-dvservices.org.au/about/our-counselling-services

Rape & Domestic Violence Services Australia (R&DVSA). (2019c). Our history. Retrieved from www.rape-dvservices.org.au/about/our-history

Rape & Domestic Violence Services Australia (R&DVSA). (2019d). Our supporters. Retrieved from https://www.rape-dvservices.org.au/about/our-supporters

Rape & Domestic Violence Services Australia (R&DVSA). (2019e) Student placements. Retrieved from www.rape-dvservices.org.au/careers/student-placements

Reavey, P. (2003). When past meets present to produce a sexual 'other'. Examining professional and everyday narratives of child sexual abuse and sexuality. In P. Reavey & S. Warner (Eds.), *New feminist stories of child sexual abuse: Sexual scripts and dangerous dialogues* (pp. 148–166). London, UK: Routledge.

Reavey, P., & Brown, S. D. (2007). Rethinking agency in memory: Space and embodiment in memories of child sexual abuse. *Journal of Social Work Practice, 21*(1), 5–21.

Rose, N. (1996). Critical history and psychology. In C. F. Graumann & K. J. Gergen (Eds.), *Historical dimensions of psychological discourse.* New York, NY: Cambridge University Press.

Rose, N., O'Malley, P., & Valverde, M. (2009). Governmentality. *Annual Review of Law and Social Science, 2*, 83–104.

Rosebank. (2019). Annual report 2018–2019. Retrieved from www.rosebank.org.au/about-us/annual-reports/

Roy, S. (2009). Melancholic politics and the politics of melancholia: The Indian women's movement. *Feminist Theory, 10*(3), 341–357.

Roy, S. (2011). Politics, passion and professionalization in contemporary Indian feminism. *Sociology, 54*(4), 587–602. https://doi.org/10.1177/0038038511406584

Royal Commission into Institutional Responses to Child Sexual Abuse. (2017). Final report. Our inquiry, Commonwealth of Australia www.childabuseroyalcommission.gov.au/sites/default/files/final_report_-_volume_1_our_inquiry.pdf

Russell, D. E. H. (1982). *Rape in marriage*. New York, NY: Macmillan.

Russell, D. E. H. (1984). *Sexual exploitation: Rape, child sexual abuse, and workplace harassment*. Beverly Hills, California: Sage.

SA Health. (2019). Yarrow Place. Retrieved from www.sahealth.sa.gov.au/wps/wcm/connect/public+content/sa+health+internet/health+services/yarrow+place+services

Sawer, M. (1990). *Sisters in suits. Women and public policy in Australia*. North Sydney, Australia: Allen & Unwin.

Sawicki, J. (2005). Queering Foucault and the subject of feminism. In G. Gutting (Ed.), *The Cambridge companion to Foucault* (pp. 379–399). Cambridge, UK: Cambridge University Press.

Schofield, T., & Goodwin, S. (2006). Gender politics and public policy making: Prospects for advancing gender equality. *Policy and Society, 24*(4), 25–44.

Skehill, C. (2007). Researching the history of social work: exposition of a history of the present approach. European Journal of Social Work, 10(4), 449–463.

Spongberg, M. (1998). Rape. In B. Caine (Ed.), *Australian feminism: A companion* (pp. 254–263). Melbourne, Australia: Oxford University Press.

Stark, E. (2007). *Coercive control: How men entrap women in personal life*. New York, NY: Oxford University Press.

Summers, A. (1999). *Ducks on the pond: An autobiography 1945–1976*. Ringwood, Australia: Viking.

Sydney Rape Crisis Centre (SRCC). (1994). *Annual report: 1993–1994*. Sydney, Australia: Author.

Tasmanian Government. (n.d.). Sexual assault services. Retrieved from https://www.communities.tas.gov.au/csr/information_and_resources/family_and_community_violence/sexual_assault_services

WA Government. (n.d.). Sexual assault resource centre (SARC). Retrieved from www.kemh.health.wa.gov.au/Our-services/Statewide-Services/SARC

Ward, E. (1984). *Father-daughter rape*. London, UK: The Women's Press.

Watson, J., Maylea, C., Roberts, R., Hill, N., & McCallum, S. (2020). *Preventing gender-based violence in mental health inpatient units* (Research report, 01/2020). Sydney, Australia: ANROWS.

Weeks, W. (1993). Women's contribution to community services. In J. Inglis & L. Rogan (Eds.), *Beyond swings and roundabouts* (pp. 67–79). Sydney, Australia: Pluto Press.

Weeks, W. (2002). *Cultural diversity and services against sexual violence. A report from the National Association of Services against Sexual Violence (NASASV)*. Melbourne, Australia: NASASV.

Weeks, W., & Gilmore, K. (1996). How violence against women became an issue on the national policy agenda. In T. Dalton, M. Draper, W. Weekes, & J. Wiseman (Eds.), *Making social policy in Australia* (pp. 125–150). Sydney, Australia: Allen & Unwin.

Whalley, E., & Hackett, C. (2017). Carceral feminisms: The abolitionist project and undoing dominant feminisms. *Contemporary Justice Review, 20*(4), 456–473. https://doi.org/10.1080/10282580.2017.1383762

Whittier, N. (2009). *The politics of child sexual abuse: Emotions, social movements and the state*. New York, NY: Oxford University Press.

Wilkin, L., & Hillock, S. (2014). Enhancing MSW students' efficacy in working with trauma, violence, and oppression: An integrated feminist-trauma framework for social work education. *Feminist Teacher, 24*(3), 184–206.

Wills, S. (2007). Seventies chronology part 1, 1970–1972. *Australian Feminist Studies, 22*(54), 401–407.

Wills, S. (2008). Seventies chronology part 2, 1973–1979. *Australian Feminist Studies, 23*(55), 131–153.

Women's Community Health Network WA. (2020). Sexual assault services. Retrieved from www.wchnwa.org.au/services/sexual-assault-services/

Women's Health NSW. (2020). Retrieved from https://whnsw.asn.au/about-whnsw/

Women's Health Policy Review Committee. (1985). *Women's health services in New South Wales. Final Report of the Women's Health Policy Review Committee*. Sydney, Australia: Parliament of New South Wales.

CHAPTER 3

Sexual Assault as Feminist Knowledge

Introduction

'Break the silence against sexual violence' is a refrain oft chanted at Reclaim the Night or Take Back the Night marches. More than a refrain, though, it is an important feminist concept. The ways society has systemically silenced victims and the role of feminist activism and analysis in breaking that 'silence' are central to feminist work against sexual violence. It was the concept adopted by the Sydney-based WAIC in 1984 to publicise one of the first surveys conducted on incest in Australia and the title of the subsequent report produced, *Breaking the Silence: A Report Based Upon the Findings of the Women Against Incest Phone-in Survey* (Waldby & Women Against Incest [NSW], 1985). Its enduring legacy has been captured in the titles of key texts produced about the role of Australian feminist interventions against sexual and gendered violence—for example, *Challenging Silence: Innovative Responses to Sexual and Domestic Violence* (Breckenridge & Laing, 1999) and *Subjugation and Silences: The Role of the Professions in Silencing Victims of Domestic and Sexual Violence* (Breckenridge, 1999). It

This chapter contains material reprinted from *Women's Studies International Forum*, 74 (May–June), Suzanne Egan, "Excavating feminist knowledges and practices in the field of sexual assault service provision: An Australian case study", 169–178, Copyright (2019), with permission from Elsevier.

S. Egan, *Putting Feminism to Work*,
https://doi.org/10.1007/978-3-030-22109-6_3

is important, though, to pause to consider both the historical nature of that silence and how feminism has challenged that silence.

I begin this chapter with a brief sketch of historical representations of rape from the late-nineteenth century onwards and use these representations as juxtapositions with which to illuminate the different understandings feminist analyses have brought to bear on the question of how we think about 'what sexual assault is' and the different ways this enables us to respond.

My primary aim through this chapter is to demonstrate what this feminist knowledge looks like when put to work through contemporary sexual assault service provision. Drawing on my research on Australian sexual assault service provision, I illustrate the ways key feminist ideas are embedded in the architecture of these services and enacted through the routine practices of sexual assault workers. Continuing my dialogue with current feminist debates about the place of feminism in contemporary work against sexual assault, I aim to problematise the 'perils of institutionalisation' narrative in which the incorporation of sexual assault organisations into the funding and regulatory processes of the state is equated with the loss of feminist political activism and commitment to social change. As discussed in Chapter 2, the services in which I conducted my research very much exemplify the key characteristics of institutionalised services. They are either government or government-funded services, professionalised (staffed by professionally qualified and trained workers), which focus on work with individual victims and routinely engage with law, police and medical systems. Yet rather than being in decline, feminism holds the type of authority that has enabled it to become the accepted, commonplace understanding of sexual violence, an understanding that has been written into the fabric of service provision.

Historical Understandings of Rape

The purported association between mental instability and women's accounts of sexual violence has a long though evolving history. In nineteenth-century medicine, hysteria was a condition believed to cause women to make false accusations of rape. 'Paranoid' middle-aged women were similarly believed prone to develop false notions of sexual violation. As Joanna Bourke (2012) in her analysis of UK and US medical texts of that time points out, such 'fabrications' would become part of the evidence used to diagnose the patient's insanity. A prominent medical jurisprudence text of the 1830s, for example, cites a case in which a young woman found near death as a result of an apparent gang rape was nevertheless found to be an 'imposter' on account of the state of 'hysteria' in which she was found. Rather than reactions to the *experience* of rape, expressions of emotional or psychological distress—'hysteria'—were used as evidence of the *fabrication* of that experience.

Contributing to, if not underpinning, such routine dismissal was the belief that it was physically impossible for a man to rape a woman who resisted his 'advances' (Bourke, 2012). Textbooks on medical jurisprudence used in this period, for example, proffered by way of analogy the impossibility of sheathing a sword in a 'vibrating scabbard' (Stoer, 1868, cited in Bourke, 2012, p. 34). One of the few circumstances where women's accounts were accorded legitimacy was when they were rendered 'insensible' during the attack. Appearing frequently in both popular and forensic accounts of rape during the nineteenth century, the condition refers to a physical rather than a psychological reaction. The victim may, for example, have fainted, had a fever or in some other way been rendered not quite 'sensible', and because of this was unable to physically resist her attacker. In keeping with the belief about the physical impossibility of raping a resisting woman, the condition of 'insensibility' rendered the woman's account legitimate and meant that her moral virtue remained intact, as she had been physically incapable of protecting her honour and chastity (Bourke, 2012).

By the 1920s, the work of Havelock Ellis, considered the leading authority on sexual behaviour, was used to justify men's right to access women's bodies in the guise of scientific objectivity and sexual liberalism. His key works are centred on the premise that 'normal' heterosexual sex is based in biologically determined power relationships in which male domination and female submission are not just inevitable but necessary for sexual pleasure (Preston, 2014). In contrast to the Victorian era view that 'normal' women were without sexual desire, Ellis believed women possessed a 'spontaneous' form of sexual impulse that manifests in a desire to be dominated. Force and therefore a degree of pain came to be understood as a normal part of heterosexual courtship rituals and as necessary to ensure women experience sexual pleasure (Preston, 2014). Consequently, signs of resistance can be interpreted as pretence or as part of a woman's sexual urge to be conquered. The 'science of sex' provided a justification for a type of biologically determined male sexuality based on power and violence. As Andrea Dworkin (1981) highlights, Ellis's work played a key role in normalising male sexual violence: Women enjoy forced sex, and men have a natural urge to do so. Indeed, his influence extended to the popular as well as professional realm, with his ideas forming the prototype for numerous marriage manuals produced in the mid-twentieth century (p. 16). Evan as late as the 1970s, Diana Russell (1984) in her analysis of the literature prior to undertaking the first US sexual assault prevalence study discovered the dominant view in the professional clinical literature was that women enjoyed the experience of rape.

The few early social science researchers working in the area mirrored these types of victim-blaming beliefs (Gavey, 2019, p. 28). For example, in mid-twentieth-century United States, Menachem Amir (1968), based on analysis of rape cases that had been reported to police in Philadelphia, developed his concept of 'victim precipitated rape'. Contrary to popular belief that the violent stranger posed most danger to women, Amir found that many of the victims knew their attacker. Rather than subject the rapists' behaviour in this cohort to analysis, Amir focused on the victims, identifying a significant subset where he believed the victim had behaved in a way that 'precipitated' the rape. Such behaviours included 'seductive' behaviour by the victim, alcohol consumption and wearing 'revealing' clothing. Amir's concept of 'victim precipitation' rests on the assumption—and his hypothesis—that if the victim does not conform to accepted 'feminine' standards of behaviour or appearance, the perpetrator will in their mind consider their actions justified—the victim deserved it. Similarly, Eugene Kanin (1957, 1969), in research he conducted on dating and courtship relationships, concluded that it was reasonable to expect some women played a provocative and sexually receptive role in the levels of male aggression identified in the study. Rather than subjecting the apparent 'normalcy' of male aggression in intimate relationships to theoretical analysis, Kanin theorised the victim as 'sexual provocateur'.

As Gavey (2019) highlights, the standard understanding of rape in the mid-twentieth century was one where rape was romanticised as a 'crime of passion'. Unless committed by a stranger, rape could easily be accommodated within accepted understandings of heterosexuality—that is, 'just sex'. When understood as motivated by a man's frustrated sexual needs, and when those 'normal' means are thwarted, rape becomes an understandable response. In this understanding, the assumed qualities of women's sexuality could be used to hold her responsible: Her body, her sexuality, provoked the attack (p. 30).

Feminist Interventions

Against this backdrop, the analytical work of second-wave feminists represents a profound intervention into contemporary understandings of rape and sexual violence. Focusing on the experience of victims, feminists argued that rape was not 'sex gone wrong' but a criminal act of violence. In the words of early theorist Susan Griffin (1977), 'Rape is an act of aggression in which the victim is denied her self-determination. It is an act of violence' (p. 66). The reformulation of rape as being about violence and not sex represents one of the key shifts in meaning attributable to second-wave feminist activism and scholarship (Gavey, 2019; Mason, 2002). It has enabled a move towards seeing rape from the woman's point of view as a degrading and disempowering experience and a set of conceptual tools through which responsibility shifts from the victim to the offender. Importantly, it is a framework that, while acknowledging sexual violence is perpetrated by one individual (usually a male) on another (usually a female), locates those individual acts of violence within a broader social, political and community context of structural power and gender inequality.

These types of feminist ideas, which in some ways could now be considered 'generic', are founded in radical feminist analyses of sexual violence, often represented as having contributed most to feminist theorising of violence against women (Bell, 1993; Carmody, 2000; Irwin, 2004; Jackson, 1996; Mason, 2002). Edwards (1987) provides a useful account of the shifts and changes over time within radical feminist theories, particularly changes in the relationship between male violence and women's oppression. Earlier radical feminists, such as Firestone (1970) and Millett (1970), theorised male dominance as vested in a range of institutions—social, political, economic and ideological—so that while male violence was positioned as part of this dominance, it was not accorded the key role characteristic of later work.

In later theories, which Edwards (1987) refers to as feminist analyses of male violence, violence against women is positioned as central to the production and maintenance of patriarchal power and therefore the key source of women's oppression. Initial texts such as Brownmiller (1975) and Griffin (1977) focused on particular forms of violence such as rape, but over time, theorists such as Dworkin (1982), McKinnon (1982, 1983) and Rich (1980) developed analyses encompassing all forms of violence, abuse and exploitation and positioned them within a patriarchal, male-dominated system. In these frameworks, the institution of heterosexuality becomes central to understanding women's oppression.

Whereas Brownmiller (1975) identified rape or the threat of it as the means through which all men controlled all women, theorists such as McKinnon (1982, 1983) extended the concept of violence to include pornography, sexual harassment and prostitution and analysed them as acts that legitimised aggressive male sexuality. McKinnon (1982, 1983) argued the social requirement of heterosexuality institutionalised male dominance and female passivity and identified sexuality as the primary sphere of male power, the site at which both power and violence converge. Sexual violence is thus situated within the context of normative heterosexuality, where aggressive male sexuality as the accepted norm is enacted through a variety of linked behaviours from sexually harassing women through to committing acts of sexual assault. Consequently, sexual relationships between men and women are characterised as inherently coercive, leading McKinnon to question whether rape could be distinguished from sex under conditions of male dominance.

Despite some nuanced differences, these analyses of male violence share a common conceptual foundation and constitute a distinctive 'type' of theoretical work. Male violence against women, whether limited to rape or extended to pornography and sexual harassment, is located within a patriarchal power system, and it is this system that produces, legitimises and maintains male dominance and female subordination. The foundation of the concept of patriarchy is a structural understanding of power, 'the idea of power as an autonomous and fundamental social structure that produces a coherent and stable set of relations by which men have dominance over women' (Mason, 2002, p. 121). Thus, the subject speaking from a radical feminist position articulates a consistent, recognisable set of responses to the question of 'what is sexual assault?' Sexual assault is an expression of the unequal power relationships between men and women and a method for maintaining inequality in a patriarchal society.

Illuminating Feminist Knowledge and Practices in Contemporary Sexual Assault Service Provision

Contemporary sexual assault services appear qualitatively different from the 'archetypical' feminist collective of the 1970s and 1980s, which operated from an explicitly feminist politics (e.g. Burke, 1992; Carmody, 1995;

Jones & Cook, 2008). Indeed, in the field of service provision in which I conducted my study, the term 'feminist' often did not appear in the types of documents (policy manuals, job advertisements, employment documents, website material and service brochures) that establish the formal apparatus of a service. In many ways, these services exemplify characteristics identified in the literature as indicative of the depoliticisation of sexual violence and decline in feminist influence. They are professionalised (Mardorossian, 2002; Marecek, 1999), subject to the regulatory processes of government (Bumiller, 2008) and very much concerned with interventions that focus on the individual (Burstow, 2005; Cvetkovich, 2003; Lamb, 1999; Stark, 2007).

Yet I suggest that feminist politics is visible in knowledge/practices of the sexual assault services sector. The basic feminist tenets of what sexual assault is and why it happens are embedded in the foundations of the sexual assault service, providing the logic for the bureaucratic protocol-driven rules of engagement and principles of service delivery. Take, for example, the *NSW Health Sexual Assault Policy and Procedure Manual* (NSW Health, 2005), a core programmatic document. It lays out the basic elements of NSW Health sexual assault services, including criteria for service, the principles that guide service delivery and requirements about specific practices and interventions.[1] The following excerpt leads into a section outlining the principles for working with victims of sexual assault. It is titled, simply, 'The nature of sexual assault':

> Sexual assault is a crime for which the offender is solely responsible. It is commonly perpetrated by someone known to the victim. Sexual assault is an act of coercion that is frequently experienced by the victim as life threatening. Whether or not injuries occur, sexual assault is an act of violence. Some offenders use their positions of power or authority to assault those whom they can readily control, such as individuals with an intellectual disability. In the majority of cases, the offenders of sexual assault are men. Prevailing community attitudes and denial about sexual assault can exacerbate the shame and self-blame that victims experience, and act as barriers to effective reporting and policing of sexual violence. Although the majority of victims

[1] This policy underpinned and guided service interventions from 2005 until early 2020. The understanding of the nature of sexual assault laid out in newly released edition of this policy (Responding to *Sexual assault (adult and child) policy and procedures)* remains consistent with the above.

> are women, many men also experience sexual assault as adults. (NSW Health, 2005, p. 84)

This definition of 'what sexual assault is' has the hallmarks of a feminist analysis. Sexual assault is not about frustrated male sexual needs; it is about coercion and power. Sexual assault is not an illness or about deviance; it is a crime and an act of violence. Sexual assault is not about female 'promiscuity' or 'leading him on' or any of the other beliefs—still evident in parts of the community—that apportion blame to the victim. The offender is 'solely' responsible. Although the term 'feminist' appears nowhere in the short factual definition of the 'nature' of sexual assault, nor in any part of the document, these are feminist ideas.

The brevity, a single paragraph, together with the factual nature of the account is indicative of the embedded and uncontested status feminist knowledge of sexual assault has assumed in the field. As Hall (2004) asserts, once an idea has achieved dominance, there is little need to expand, explain or defend that idea. Indeed, an identifying characteristic of discourses that have achieved the status of truth is the extent to which they are treated as 'common sense' and self-evident forms of knowledge that do not require explanation, elaboration or defence.

To illustrate by way of contrast, the explanation of the nature of sexual assault contained in a much earlier government document on sexual abuse was so extensive that it was attached in a separate appendices. This document, the *Report of the New South Wales Child Sexual Assault Task Force* (1987), produced in response to lobbying by feminists on the issue of child sexual abuse, led to the roll-out of the network of sexual assault services across NSW. Importantly, this was a document produced during the decade—the 1980s—in which recognition of the problem of 'incest' or child sexual assault was only just coming to public attention. During this period, theories such as those that attributed incest to family dysfunction were still prominent among professionals such as psychiatrists, as were contestations between feminist organisations and other groups, such as child protection advocates and psychiatrists, over who should provide services to victims (Breckenridge, 1992). Using a family dysfunction framework, for example, meant that incest was understood as symptomatic of an underlying family breakdown for which all family members were responsible and consequently all members, including the perpetrator, would be involved in the therapeutic intervention. In this context, it is not surprising that a document produced by a government-appointed taskforce and that explicitly adopted a feminist analysis of child sexual assault would require elaboration of concepts such as male power and the patriarchal nuclear family and careful explanation of the reasons for understanding child sexual assault within a feminist framework. The fact that, by the 2000s, a feminist analysis of sexual assault could be written as a brief factual statement in a core government document suggests that sexual assault has become, at least in this context, embedded feminist knowledge.

Even the most basic principle of service provision—the exclusion of the offender and the focus on the needs and experiences of the victim—is premised on a quite specific understanding of what 'sexual assault is'. A service provision model focused exclusively on the victim's needs and care requires a significant discursive shift. It requires that responsibility shifts from the victim to the offender, that the victim is believed rather than subjected to questions about their 'role' in the assault and that the experience of forced sex is understood as an act of criminal violence, not 'just sex'. In short, it requires a feminist analysis of 'what sexual assault is'.

In the contemporary context, it may seem almost 'common sense' that sexual assault services are victim services. However, even when the first services were set up in NSW in the late 1970s, this was not understood automatically. As Carmody (1995) recounts in her history of the development of the NSW sexual assault services sector, when the first centres opened, there was initial confusion among police officers over whether it was the victim or the perpetrator they should be bringing to the centres. Moreover, there are ways of understanding sexual assault that are compatible with victims and perpetrators sharing the service space. If, within sexual assault services, child sexual assault were positioned as a problem of family dysfunction, the rules of engagement would be different. The service would engage with both victim and abuser. However, as Breckenridge (1992) points out, the 'family dysfunction' discourse was explicitly rejected in the taskforce report that guided the roll-out of sexual assault services across NSW. Perhaps a legacy of this rejection can still be seen in current service brochures and policy manuals that consistently specify that only 'non-offending family members' can access services.

Mobilising Feminist Knowledge Through Worker Practices

Analysis of worker practices provides a more nuanced account of how the 'truth status' of feminism operates in the field of sexual assault and provides insight into what abstract ideas, theories and policies 'look like' when they are put to work in individuals' practices. In this section, I lay out the typical ways practitioners mobilise feminist concepts to produce a recognisable set of 'truth' statements about sexual assault. In the final part of the chapter, I lay out how these concepts articulate into a set of recognisably feminist practices.

Sexual assault is about gender, about power and about violence. The following excerpts are illustrative both of the repetitive pattern in which these concepts occur and of the ways they are deployed to build a narrative account about the problem of sexual violence. Knitted together through the 30 practitioner interviews, sexual assault is consistently presented as an act that, while committed by an individual, is located within and symptomatic of a system of gendered inequality that advantages men (as a category) and disadvantages women and children.

> I guess I do a traditional feminist analysis, which—I mean, it's a gender analysis, it's a power analysis. I see the causes as rooted in the ability for people, and often gender-wise it's men, to exploit their relative power in our community so that the power of children and women is less so and their avenues of recourse to it less so Like, it's a social issue, the causes are social because in our society the way in which masculinity is constructed allows for relatively normal men to do it because the consequences that are attached to doing it don't seem to be that severe either. Often non-existent. (Interview Text No. 8)

> It's using a position of privilege and power and trust to violate and abuse and that it's a person usually a male making a choice—to do the wrong thing—and to use this position of power to abuse. I think while the individual offender is always responsible and makes a choice to abuse, society still has a fairly high level of denial about child sexual assault which contributes to the silence around it that only ever supports an offender. (Interview Text No. 16)

> [It is] the kind of privilege that is usually afforded to men in relationships and in the world, yeah. Like socially and politically. Yeah. And the kind of

> entitlement that then comes with that privilege and the ideas and the actions that come out of that provide an opportunity for violent type behaviour to flourish. (Interview Text No. 9)

In each of these excerpts, the practitioners' understanding of sexual violence consistently moves between the focus on the individual offender's abuse of power, their responsibility for that abuse and the positioning of those individual acts within broader systems of gendered social inequality. In these narratives, attribution of responsibility to the offender is enabled by a clear conceptual linking of structural power and the individual power offenders use to perpetrate sexual violence. Sexual assault offenders use their socially sanctioned position of power and privilege to abuse women and children. They are not misfits but 'relatively normal men' whose actions are largely supported by community denial and who experience little in the way of consequences because of how their behaviour is normalised. In this context, it is important to stress, as the practitioners do, the offender's criminal responsibility, to be clear that sexual assault is not just a sexual encounter gone wrong but an act of criminal violence (Gavey, 2019). This constructs the legal identity not only of the offender but also, by implication, the victim.

Some feminist scholars have been critical of what they see as an over-involvement by feminists working against sexual violence on legal redress and criminal action at the expense of work that focuses on broad-based social change (Bumiller, 2008), including access to state-based services being dependent on police involvement (Jones & Cook, 2008). The criminality of sexual assault is foundational to the field of NSW sexual assault service provision as indeed it is in sexual assault services across all Australian states and territories. This not only clearly positions the offender as outside the remit of the sexual assault service and within the jurisdiction of the criminal justice system, but also means that services engage with clients on the premise that they are victims of crime.

Sexual assault counsellors routinely interact with the legal system, accompanying victims to court, providing resources and information about the legal process and liaising with police and lawyers.[2] Moreover,

[2] There are some similarities between this role and that of the UKs Independent Sexual Violence Advisers (ISVA) who are located in either the government Sexual Assault Referral Services or the voluntary sector rape crisis Centres, and whose role is to provide advocacy and support tailored to victims needs as victims of crime (Hester & Lilley, 2017; Robinson & Hudson, 2011). However unlike the UK model, court support, preparation and advocacy

services continue to play an active and important role in law reform, through membership of both state- and local-level committees that convene around the issues of legal reform and the implementation of current law. An example of the type of reform achieved is that both child and adult victims now give their evidence in court via CCTV, with a support person, usually a sexual assault worker, present so they do not have to see the accused offender. In NSW, the video-recorded police statement of child witnesses is played in court as their 'evidence in chief' with the aim of reducing the number of times the child has to recount distressing details. More recently, R&DVSA, an organisation with a long history of advocating for victim-centred legal reforms, made the landmark decision to employ a legal officer. Having long been at the forefront of campaigns for victim-focused legal reforms, the creation of this new position has significantly strengthened the organisation's capacity to influence a range of recent state and national legal inquiries and reviews, including consent in relation to sexual offences in NSW (R&DVSA, 2019a; 2019c), non-consensual sharing of intimate images (R&DVSA, 2018b), changes to police powers (R&DVSA, 2019b) and to the Australian family law system (R&DVSA, 2018a).

However, while services are involved in legal reform, and counsellors do provide support to victims who pursue legal action, reporting the crime to the police is not a requirement of victims seeking assistance from sexual assault services.[3] As the following excerpt from the NSW Health sexual

work is the part of the role of all counsellors in sexual assault services. Moreover the focus of the ISVAS on the criminal response to sexual assault suggests these positions may have more in common with the Witness Assistance Service, which is a support service provided by the public prosecutor's office (NSW Office of the Department of Public Prosecutions) to all victims of crime who are involved in criminal proceedings.

[3] Nor is the person required to provide details of their abuse or have the information they provide verified in order to access counselling and support. This is in contrast to generic victims of crime services. For example, the application process for the Approved Counselling Service (ACS) provided through the NSW Department of Communities and Justice to victims of violent crimes requires the applicant to provide specific details (such as exact location and address) of the assault and, if reported, the name of the police or organisation. The applicant's details are then verified as part of the application process, and supporting documentation can be requested (NSW Department of Communities and Justice, n.d.). In addition, while the legislative framework of the service no longer requires the victim to have made a police report (Victims Rights and Support Act 2013 [NSW Government, 2013]), the promotional material maintains a focus on support through the 'justice journey'—that is, the journey criminal legal proceedings process (NSW Department of Communities and Justice, n.d.)

assault policy makes explicit, it is the victim's decision whether to report the assault to the police:

> The decision to proceed with a formal complaint to the police rests with the victim, and the service is to respect the victim's wishes ... counsellors are not required to report sexual assault to police if this is against a client's wishes. (NSW Health, 2005, p. 15)

It is thus clear that choice in relation to criminal justice action is important:

> Although sexual assault is a crime, it should always remain the choice of the victim as to whether they proceed with a formal complaint to police ... Workers are required to provide clear information in an unbiased manner to assist victims to decide whether it is in their interests to proceed with a formal complaint. (NSW Health, 2005, p. 84)

Nor are the services involved in the work of criminal investigation, which is clearly delineated as the NSW police's role (NSW Health, 2005). Rather, the sexual assault worker's role is an advocate who supports the victim as she comes to her own decision about whether to make a police report, whether to have the forensic medical examination or, further down the track, whether to continue with a court case.

This stance extends to situations where counsellors and medical practitioners are present at, or involved in, interventions pertinent to criminal investigation. The next extract, from the NSW Health policy, concerns the role of the medical practitioners who examine victims of sexual assault, often to collect 'forensic' evidence of the assault from the victim's body or clothing. The policy states that although

> in some cases, information from the medical examination can assist the investigation of allegations of abuse and contribute to prosecution of offenders ... in all cases they [medical practitioners] have an important role to play in identifying medical treatment needs and providing support and reassurance. (NSW Health, 2005, p. 3)

As the policy states, performing medical examinations to collect evidence for criminal investigation 'may, in some cases' assist in the investigation and prosecution of the offender. However, it should never be the only or even primary role of the medical practitioner. As the policy goes on to spell out, regardless of whether or not a forensic medical examination is performed, *all* medical practitioners have an important role in 'providing support and reassurance' to victims and in identifying where they may have medical needs that require treatment. Examples of these types of medical treatment can include prescribing the morning after pill in assaults where there is risk of pregnancy, testing for sexually transmitted infections (STIs) or prescribing prophylactics.[4]

It is important at this point to highlight the extent to which the medical response is an integrated part of the service provided by NSW Health sexual assault services.[5] At the broader policy and training level, this integration is reflected in the medical and forensic training and resources provided by the ECAV,[6] the training body that as discussed oversees all key professional development training for sexual assault workers employed in the government (health) sector. At the service level, this integration means the coordinator has responsibility for coordinating medical care as well as the crisis counselling response and has oversight of training for and supervision of staff, including collaborative input into medical staff training on matters related to sexual assault (NSW Health, 2005, p. 50). For example,

[4] These key points about the place of the medical examination and role of the police remains constant in the updated Policy Responding to *Sexual assault (adult and child) policy and procedures* (*2020*). Indeed, in some respects the stance has been strengthened. For example the policy provides and explicit rationale for medical examinations taking place in a health rather than a justice environment and conceptualises any collection of forensic evidence as an 'adjunct' to the care provided to the victim—in those instances where they may wish to pursue legal action. Thus a medical response remains part of an integrated crisis response where interventions are guided by the wishes of the person and centre on their health safety and wellbeing (NSW Health, 2020, p. 94).

[5] This integrated response shares some similarities with the government based sexual assault referral centre (SARCs) introduced in the UK from the early 2000s (Hester & Lilley, 2017) in that both models aim to promote an integrated response by the systems involved in responding to sexual assault. However, while the NSW services do work closely with a number of other systems (such as legal and police) they are not structured on the 'one stop shop' model of SARCs in which staff seconded from health (doctors to perform forensic medicals), specialist police (sexual offences liaison officers) Independent Sexual Violence Advisers (ISVA) and counsellors all form part of the specialist sexual assault referral centres (Robinson & Hudson, 2011). Rather the NSW service model (like other Australian states and territories) is based on protocols and agreements between the specialist sexual assault services and other systems such as police and the broader health system.

[6] Examples include the Graduate Certificate in Medical & Forensic Management of Adult Sexual Assault, a shorter medical examiner 'update' style workshops and written resources such as a practice manual (ECAV, n.d.-a).

the service coordinator typically has oversight of the crisis roster, ensuring that each shift is staffed by both an on-call counsellor and medical practitioner. This responsibility flows into the crisis counsellor's work who is 'responsible within the service for coordinating the overall care of the client and the assessment of their social and emotional needs' (NSW Health, 2005, p. 28). This means that a medical examination is not to take place before the counsellor has met with the victim in order to ascertain those needs and importantly to provide the information the person may need to make decisions about the medical examination (NSW Health, 2005, p. 28). Often, the counsellor will be present at the examination to both witness the examination and provide support to the victim.

Certainly, during the time I worked as a sexual assault counsellor, I supported many victims, both child and adult, during their medical examinations. My observation and experience are that the counsellor does play an important role in the crisis and medical response. It is important, for example, to be able to explain to people what happens during and after a medical examination. It is important for people to know they can have a forensic examination but withhold permission for it to be released to the police until after they have had time to decide if they want to take legal action. Likewise, it is important, especially when working with children, to make sure they understand and agree to the examination and that their parents or carers are able to understand that the purpose of the examination is not to 'prove' the abuse occurred. Mostly, I think it is important that counsellors and medical examiners are able to work collaboratively to ensure that the person is given the best possible response in what is usually a highly distressing and sometimes overwhelming situation.

In making this point, I am not trying to assert that every such crisis and medical response occurs in a seamlessly collaborative manner, and I am certainly not intending to negate victims' experiences where a poor medical, police or counselling response has added to rather than helped alleviate their distress. What I am suggesting is that it is possible to do so in a manner that does not automatically equate to depoliticisation or indicate a dissipation of feminist influence.

Feminism can be about public protest. It can also be about working with the systems that respond to sexual violence and assisting women to negotiate those complex and still very inequitable systems. Moreover, the catalyst for reform often comes from individuals' experiences and the detailed knowledge accumulated by counsellors and services through their interactions with individual police officers, prosecutors and medical practitioners; the policies and procedures governing those interactions, together with their clients' experiences, play an important role in wider change. In both instances, the aim is to intervene to try to reduce further distress and victimisation and to ensure the system becomes more responsive to the needs and rights of victims and survivors.

Producing Feminist Counselling Techniques

NSW sexual assault services are involved in broader responses to sexual violence (community development, community education and prevention programmes and, as I have just discussed, legal reform). Indeed, to be considered a sexual assault service within the NSW Health system, services are required to have some involvement in prevention and community education work. Counselling is, however, the primary work and type of intervention provided by both NGO and government services. It is the intervention highlighted in service brochures, the essential skill cited in job advertisements and the focus of professional skills development. For example, the overwhelming majority of sexual assault training workshops offered by the ECAV focus primarily on counselling and therapeutic skills development.[7] Perhaps not surprisingly, this focus was reflected in the career trajectories of the participants in my study, most of whom had come to work in the sexual assault services sector from casework and counselling positions in areas such as domestic violence services, child protection and women's health services. None, for example, had come from positions where their work had focused on working with communities (community development), facilitating groups or providing community-based education programmes. Moreover, accounts of their counselling and therapeutic work dominated the practitioner interviews, including in the examples of practice models and interventions that were given to demonstrate how their knowledge of the causes and consequences of sexual violence played out in their day-to-day work.

Three core feminist counselling techniques were identifiable in the practitioner texts: techniques that work with the concept of power, techniques that focus on self-blame and techniques that focus on the

[7] Examples from the courses offered by ECAV include 'Advanced therapeutic work with adult survivors of child sexual abuse', 'Therapeutic practices with children, young people and adults affected by shame', and 'Therapeutic responses to children, young people and adults with an intellectual disability who have been sexually abused (ECAV, n.d.-b).

relationship between the individual and the structures that support sexual assault. Each technique made visible the ways practitioners mobilised their broad conceptual or theoretical understandings of sexual violence and put them to work to guide their interactions with victims and survivors. As this practitioner explained, understanding 'sexual violence as a gendered crime', coupled with a broader feminist analysis of 'the way the world works', influenced how she viewed her role, whether it be in the (often) medico–legal crisis setting or in the more therapeutically orientated ongoing counselling work:

> Well I think because having that analysis that sexual violence is a gendered crime, I think with that comes a feminist analysis of the way the world works and I think holding the principles of feminism as I see it in terms of empowering women—although they can't feel more powerless than experiencing sexual violence, so obviously I'm in the role of trying to facilitate that power for them—maximising choice. I kind of hold that pretty much in feminism. And I would—that's the way I work, in terms, you know, whether it's in the crisis setting or my own counselling with people, it's impacting people's choices, trying to give that power back. (Interview Text No. 7)

Working with Power

Power, or the abuse of power inherent in sexual assault, is the linchpin in the production of a specifically feminist counselling practice in this field. The conceptual or theoretical understanding of sexual assault as an abuse of power articulates into practices that focus on enabling and supporting victims to make their own choices and decisions, on collaborative practices and on the victim regaining power as a strategy to recover from the experience of sexual assault. As this practitioner highlighted, 'because sexual assault is about power and control [it is] essential to recovery to give the person their power back. So they must control their recovery; they must be making their own decisions' (Interview Text No. 1).

This understanding of sexual victimisation as an experience disempowers women who produce counselling practices that focus on how power is practised within the counselling relationship, as this excerpt illustrates:

> Empowering people to feel that sense of control over their own lives again. That also fundamentally guides what I do and the way I practise. And that empowerment approach also has a feminist base in that you're not wanting to have more power than the client.

> You're wanting to be—the role of expert can be another example of the way power is being used against someone. So not wanting to do that. Wanting to be working from a more collaborative approach. (Interview Text No. 29)

Eschewing 'the role of expert' in favour of collaborative practices that facilitate women's choice and autonomy has a long history in feminist work against male violence. As discussed, it was key to the development by second-wave feminists of individual and collective practices designed to challenge and provide alternatives to the hierarchical power structures associated with mainstream patriarchal institutions (Jones & Cook, 2008; Weeks, 1993).

This principle underpins the crisis counsellor's crucial role in working with and advocating for the victim/survivor to ensure they have the time, space and information they need to decide whether to undergo a medical examination, or whether they will make a police statement, or later down the track continue with court proceedings. This type of practice, this appreciation of the subtleties of power and power dynamics, requires sensitivity and nuance. It means keeping the survivor and her needs, decisions and wishes at the centre of the interaction while also acknowledging and allowing space for the reactions and concerns of parents and family members who are often enormously impacted.

For example, in the next excerpt, a counsellor provides insight into how she negotiated this space with the family who were concerned that their daughter, who had been sexually victimised by a work colleague, had decided she did not want to be involved in criminal proceedings. In particular, they were worried their daughter may later regret 'that she never did anything about it' and wondered if they should try to persuade her to change her mind. As the counsellor explains below, while not discounting their concerns and worries, she emphasised the positive ongoing effects on the young woman of knowing that her parents had supported her choice.

> 'Well, you know, she may do that but what she will remember is that you supported her and her decisions and when she has to make difficult decisions in the future, she will know that you are a source of support'. And that's what's important. That you support her in her choices and decisions. So, you know, that's feminist practice. (Interview Text No. 20)

And as the counsellor pointed out, this is 'feminist practice'. It is an example of taking what could be, and is sometimes, read as an abstract set of theoretical principles and ideas and using them to guide everyday individual encounters and interventions.

While the contemporary service may look different from those original collectively organised centres of the late 1970s and 1980s, the centrality of working differently with power has not only survived the incorporation of the services into the state's governance structures, but has also been written into the policies, procedures and practices that govern the sector. This principle underpins the policies that say it is the victim's choice about whether to report to the police or undergo a medical examination, and it clearly removes the sexual assault service from any investigative role, thus enabling them to work with and ensure they have the resources to make their own decision.

Working with Self-Blame

Self-blame, the tendency of victims to hold themselves responsible for the sexual assault, was consistently cited across the library of documents (service brochures, interview texts, information booklets for victims, service manuals, and policy and procedure manuals) as one of the primary effects of sexual assault. In much of the research literature on sexual assault, self-blame is theorised as psychological in origin, as a cognitive deficit characteristic of abuse victims (McCann & Pearlman, 1990) or as having a regressive character 'congruent with the thought processes of early childhood, in which the self is taken as the reference point for all events' (Herman, 1997, p. 103). However, as the following excerpts illustrate, self-blame was positioned through the interview texts in a way that 'normalised', rather than pathologised, victims.

> But you know, just seeing them even the next day or very soon after, there's that whole thing about 'but it was my fault' and so the self-blame and just the total effects that has on a lot of women. Some women if they've got good social supports and that, and good networks, and depending on their personalities or just where they're coming from in their belief systems tend to fare a lot better than some other women. But a lot of women, I'd say, even those that have the best support systems, there's always an element of self-blame. 'If only I had' or 'I shouldn't have', and there's definitely that sort of mantra that comes through. (Interview Text No. 10)

> Some of the universal things that I often find with sexual assault is that sense of 'there must have been something about me that made this happen. There must have been something that I did or something about me or the way I look or'—that turning the blame on yourself that seems to be universal—the ramifications of that—that can grow into just something—you know, permeates so many other parts of someone's life really… And you just see for even the most confident of people, that sense of self being eroded over time, … their confidence in their work place or in their relationships—they're second-guessing themselves constantly is just such a tragedy, I think. Given that this is something they didn't ask for, didn't want. (Interview Text No. 23)

This 'normalising' of self-blame as something most victims experience regardless of their external supports, their self-confidence or internal resources helps position this effect as a consequence of sexual victimisation rather than as attributable to personal vulnerability or pre-existing life situation.

Moreover, linking this normalised and expected consequence to broader cultural practices and societal beliefs helps produce the recursive relationship between individual experience and broader social structures and inequities (the personal as political) that lies at the heart of feminist analyses of sexual violence (e.g. Brownmiller, 1975; Griffin, 1977). The following excerpt lays out how these links are typically understood.

> I just think from their own belief systems that—that whole thing of, you know, a bloke can go out looking pretty sort of snazzy and that's okay, but if a woman goes out, you know [she's] in colloquial terms a 'slut' or something like that or easy prey and so a lot of women I think take that on board and think 'well okay, because I did this I must be somehow less worthy'. And the socialisation of women or children—or female children—is quite different to the socialisation of boys. (Interview Text No. 10)

This internalisation of societal sexual double standards through gendered socialisation practices, coupled with still-prevalent community beliefs, enables women to be placed in a position in which they (and others) hold themselves responsible. In addition, women are generally socialised in ways that position them as responsible for relationships, as this practitioner explains:

> I think generally women are trained to take responsibility for relationships. And so I think there's this kind of belief that 'I should—I could have done something to prevent that—I could have protested, I could have resisted, I could have'. There's this real kind of responsibility for them about they could have done something to prevent it happening. (Interview Text No. 7)

Here the practitioner lays out the ways broad-based heteronormative beliefs and practices articulate into a particular set of beliefs, which position the victim as responsible for the assault. While, as the excerpt indicates, this is an important factor in all forms of sexual assault, it has particular impact where the perpetrator is known to the victim, which is the case with most instances of sexual assault (Australian Bureau of Statistics, 2012).

This conceptual understanding of and knowledge about the relationship between self-blame and sexual violence produces quite concrete practices or techniques for working with this effect, as the practitioner from Interview Text No. 7 elaborates:

> I think the way I've seen it work quite well is to look [at] how—what individually they're holding in terms of blaming themselves. So I might have a whiteboard—why do you blame yourself? Not judging it—'just because this, because I wore that, because I had a drink with him'—you know, all the things that come in. So it's kind of like all the myths, really, around sexual violence come out. And then it's about dispelling them and then look at it—why do you think they're there? Who benefits from that view that you hold? So looking at how it impacts them individually and then bring it out to wider society. It alleviates their blame—you can see that the people who are benefitting are not women. It's not her. Yeah. It's the people who get away with it. (Interview Text No. 7)

This example demonstrates the skilful navigation required to move back and forth between the individual and the broader social context. The shifting of responsibility from victim to perpetrator that happens at the end of the intervention ('It's the people who get away with it' who benefit) is not a simple relocation of responsibility from one individual (the victim) to another (the offender), but comes via an exploration that implicitly situates sexual violence within a broader system of gender inequality. Evident throughout is the respectful way this technique is used, in the sense of collaborating with the client, hearing rather than dismissing their beliefs and posing careful questions that allow the client to play an active part in the process rather than having 'expert' knowledge imposed upon them. This type of practice requires not only a keen understanding of relational power inequalities but also a clear understanding of the social and cultural beliefs about women that promote sexual violence and, importantly, the capacity to translate that into enabling practices with victims and survivors.

Working Between Individuals and Structures

Counselling has been the subject of some debate within second-wave feminism, and some feminists have been critical of this type of intervention, arguing that it reduces sexual assault to an individual problem (Crook, 2018; Kitzinger, 1997). However, as Bondi (2006) points out, counselling, like feminism, is diverse and contains both 'possibilities for, and closures against, the expression of feminist commitments' (p. 347). It is important to distinguish between working with individuals and 'individualising' a social or political problem (Egan, 2019). Sexual assault practitioners do work primarily with individuals—it is a key organising principle of this field of work. However, they do so in a manner that requires they simultaneously hold a political lens to the problem of sexual assault and intervene where politics affects at the most local level, in the embodied form of individual victims/survivors. This is evident in the sensitivity to the power dynamics in the counselling relationship, in the focus on enabling the victim/survivor to regain a sense of power and control, and in the framework used to work with the complexities of self-blame.

It is also evident in the awareness of the ways the structural articulates into and shapes specific situations and experiences of the individuals with whom they work. The following excerpt exemplifies this stance.

> If you take a step back from all your clients, you will find some endemic structural abuses that support that sexual assault in every case you're working on. And you have a choice of how you respond to those. Whether it's a poor police response—whether it's how their mother views it, you know, 'you little slut', or, you know, there's something endemic around from society that supports that. (Interview Text No. 20)

This linking or situating the individual within the structural may, as in the above example, take the form of advocacy work with the police involved. It may mean working with a young person's parents to assist them in coming to understand the many societal myths and misbeliefs that may have shaped their initial responses to their child's disclosure of their abuse. For example, in the scenario I discussed in the 'Working with Power' section, while the young woman had decided she did not want to be involved in criminal action against the work colleague who had assaulted her, she did want changes in the workplace culture that she saw as enabling the assault. As a result, the sexual assault service approached the organisation and was able to work with them successfully to provide workplace sexual assault prevention education and training.

Like this example, advocacy and social change work in the sector often take place at the local level in response to local situations and occurrences. For example, another service in which I conducted interviews had begun working with local nursing homes as a response to media reports as well as referrals in relation to the sexual abuse of elderly residents in the local area. Another service located in an area known for street-based sex work worked with their local sex worker cooperative to develop a community-based outreach programme that combined informal research on how to meet the needs and increase the safety of this group along with providing support and advocacy. Some local initiatives lead into or become part of broader statewide community work. For example, a 'drink-spiking project' that began when one metropolitan service noticed a trend in increased referrals for drug-facilitated sexual assault developed into a larger project that produced a number of practical resources, such as information booklets suitable for use in services across the sector. Similarly, the work with local nursing homes has over time played an important part in the development of training programmes on the abuse of older people now provided by ECAV. In these types of initiatives, the network of statewide meetings, committees and peak bodies play an important role in enabling the tracking of trends beyond local areas and provide a mechanism for communicating local service projects and initiatives.[8]

During my own time working as a sexual assault counsellor, I was aware of and involved in a number of similar locally based projects. One such example focused on trying to make changes to our services so that it better met the needs of adolescent and young adult victims. This service was

[8] For example, staff from the NSW Health training centre (ECAV) attend the statewide meetings of NSW Health sexual assault services, which means they are able to keep track of emerging trends that may require them to add or make changes to the training programmes they provide.

located in an area with a high percentage of this population group. Yet as a service, our contact with young people who had experienced sexual violence was quite low. While some younger clients did come to the centre for counselling, others would come once or twice and not return. Given that there was a youth service close by, we sought their assistance and, during a series of meetings, talked through different possibilities for changing our service and practices. Over time, the meetings evolved into a project that focused on gaining the input of young people in the area. One of the initial ways we did this was to organise a three-day camp for young people who had experienced sexual violence. Organised jointly with the youth centre, the camp was a way we could work with the young people to get their input about the types of support and interventions they thought were important for our service to provide to young people. One of the almost immediate changes was having a sexual assault counsellor based in the youth centre on a rotating roster so that we were available to young people in the youth centre's more relaxed environment, with whom they often already had an established relationship.

These types of local interventions are important. Typically, though, they are not widely known about beyond their locale or outside the local community and service networks. There is simply not the time nor the resources to produce formal publicly available reports, much less publication pieces for academic journals, conference presentations or to publicise initiatives via media sources. At best, a document may be kept in a filing cabinet or computer file, or more likely becomes part of that institutional but unrecorded memory that is held by workers and is often lost when they leave.

Norma's Project: A Research Study Into the Sexual Assault of Older Women in Australia (Mann, Horsley, Barrett, & Tinney, 2014) provides a concrete example of what I am talking about here. Similar to the example of prevention work in local nursing homes just discussed, the research impetus was the sexual abuse of an elderly woman in an aged care facility, in this particular instance the mother of one of the researchers. As a tenured academic they—together with colleagues—were able to apply for and were successful in obtaining a three-year research grant to undertake the study, which garnered the support of a number of well-respected state and national organisations concerned with the rights of senior Australians. This was much needed and important research, and it is not my intention to detract from it. The point I want to make is that, by virtue of the report cited, conference presentations, and the other dissemination strategies available within the academy, this research has achieved a public profile in the way that local initiatives undertaken by sexual assault services generally do not. This does not mean, however, that the latter are less significant in terms of their impacts in local communities.

In some ways, the pattern or method of working by moving between the individual and the structural is not actually at its core, so it is very different from the work of the earlier sexual assault centres. As discussed in the previous chapter, the political campaigns run by SRCC, for example, often stemmed from emerging issues noted by the telephone counsellors, whether they be increasing calls from women assaulted by professionals or calls about sexual harassment and abuse on university campuses (Carmody, 1995). Similarly, during the early 1980s, data collected by the newly established government sexual assault centres on the marked increases in phone calls and referrals for child sexual abuse helped provide the impetus for campaigns designed to elicit victim and community input on the needs of and responses to victims (Carmody, 1995; Case, 1992).[9]

In particular, the NSW Sexual Assault Committee, which developed from the working party that set up the hospital-based services, provided a mechanism through which individual services could feed this information (Carmody, 1995). In turn, the Sexual Assault Committee was the primary strategy used by 'femocrats' to politicise and respond to the issue of child sexual assault (see accounts by Carmody, 1992, 1995; Franzway, Court, & Connell, 1989; Sawer, 1990). This included the statewide campaign No-one Deserves to be Raped, which involved a number of community-focused initiatives including committee members travelling to rural areas to hold public forums about sexual assault and a three-day 'phone-in' where women were encouraged to give their views on gaps in services and their suggestions for reform (Carmody, 1995). Likewise, contemporary services, whether NGO or NSW Health Sexual Assault Policy Unit, collect and analyse referral information that enables them to identify emerging issues and trends. The mechanisms for doing this are of course now quite formalised and distinctively bureaucratic. In the case of NSW Health services, for example, this includes a quite detailed form recording

[9] For example, Case (1992), drawing on her experiences at a hospital-based sexual assault centre in the early 1980s, explains that while set up as a crisis service for adults, referrals for children began to increase markedly to the extent that by the mid-1980s, they outweighed adult referrals.

de-identified information (type of assault, location, demographic details) on every client, which is collated and analysed at a state level. The collection of this type of data enables identification of trends such as increased referrals for victims of alcohol-facilitated sexual assault, for example, or can help identify what is often referred to as 'barriers' or 'gaps' in service provision. For example, if referrals to services by victims from particular demographics (e.g. age, race and ethnicity, socio-economic status, disability) are lower than the percentage of those people living in a given location, there are what is typically referred to as 'barriers' to service provision.

Despite the rather bureaucratic expression, this is an important part of the social change and social justice work undertaken in the sector. Ensuring that services are changed and provided in a way that meets the needs of all victims of sexual violence is essential to ensuring that work against sexual violence helps ameliorate rather than contribute to structural inequalities based on race, ethnicity, class, age, ability or sexuality.

I do not want to overplay the comparison. There are differences. Rather than street marches and protests, contemporary social change interventions, as outlined above, tend to be quite formalised as the examples I have provided illustrate: discrete community work projects, training workshops or via written submissions to government inquiries. Equally formalised are the relationships between services and organisations. Rather than workers gathering to form collectives or organising 'phone-ins', we have 'inter-agency' meetings, 'peak bodies' and documented 'protocols' for how to work together and form 'partnerships'. Yet, at its core, the mechanism has remained markedly stable over time—a recursive loop between work with individual victims and survivors and work at the community level, framed by the understanding that sexual assault is enabled through systemic structural inequalities.

To make a final analogy, in the late 1970s, the SRCC joined forces with the Women's Officer at one of the local universities to run a political campaign against sexual harassment and sexual abuse on campus (NSWRCC, 2008). In the contemporary context, this organisation, now known as R&DVSA, is again involved in working with universities on the issue of sexual harassment and abuse on campus.[10] In contrast to the 1970s, this is

[10] In 2016, after years of agitation by student groups, the Australian Human Rights Commission (AHRC) conducted a national survey on sexual violence experienced by students at Australian universities and in 2017 released their report *Change the Course: National Report on Sexual Abuse and Sexual Harassment at Australian Universities* (AHRC, 2017).

far from an informal grassroots initiative. Rather, the organisation is 'contracted' to run training programmes in 'partnership' with the respective organisation to educate staff and students about sexual violence. Some workshops focus on ensuring those university members identified as most likely for students to disclose incidents of sexual violence to (for example student leaders, staff of campus accommodation) have the requisite knowledge to respond to victims with empathy and understanding. Other programmes aim to prevent sexual violence by changing the attitudes, behaviours and organisational culture that enables sexual violence to occur and which ensures victims remain silent. Yet despite the formal differences (payment for services, signing of contracts, a highly educated and formally trained retinue of educators), the impetus remains the same: to ensure that victims are believed and supported and to work towards the broader systemic changes needed to eliminate sexual violence.

Conclusion

Through this chapter, I aimed to demonstrate that the individualisation and depoliticisation of a social issue such as sexual violence cannot be unproblematically equated with a particular 'type' of intervention, with a particular 'type' of worker or with a particular 'type' of service structure. If my research had 'looked' only for a particular type of service model (community based, outside the state) or a particular type of practice (grassroots activism and protest), then feminism, at best, would have registered as a much diluted and dissipated force. This is important because it not only demonstrates the robustness and adaptability of feminism but also means that the key feminist principles and concepts required to ensure victims and survivors of sexual assault are treated with dignity and respect have been incorporated into routine policies and practices. The poor treatment of victims was, after all, a major impetus for the second-wave feminist campaigns and protests.

Indeed, in this quintessentially institutionalised field of service that forms my case study, feminism has become in many ways 'mainstream', to borrow Walby's (2011) expression. In making such a statement, I am not

Because of the report's recommendations, R&DVSA, among other Australian sexual assault services, have been involved in a range of different on-campus interventions from counselling through to prevention and policy work. R&DVSA also contributed to the AHRC report and was involved with the End Rape on Campus student organisation.

trying to suggest that research based on this specific context negates issues and concerns raised about the effects of institutionalisation as that plays out across different geographies, jurisdictions and types of nation states. I am, however, suggesting that the debates, dialogues and discussions that have arisen from such concerns may be enhanced through considering both this research and what can become visible in research when feminism is approached as a form of knowledge rather than a particular 'type' of politics. Further, while some feminists (Cvetkovich, 2003; Stark, 2007) have critiqued therapeutic and counselling interventions to argue that such approaches reduce sexual victimisation to an individual problem, I countered this by highlighting the extent to which such practices can be enacted through, and indeed are dependent upon, a highly politicised analysis of sexual violence.

In the next chapter, I continue to focus on the prominence of individual interventions in contemporary service provision, turning to consider the growing dominance of 'trauma talk' in sexual assault services.

References

Amir, M. (1968). Victim precipitated forcible rape. *Journal of Criminal Law & Criminology and Police Science, 58*(4), 493–502.

Australian Bureau of Statistics. (2012). *Personal safety report.* Retrieved from http://www.abs.gov.au/ausstats/abs@.nsf/Lookup/4906.0Chapter7002012

Australian Human Rights Commission. (2017). *Change the course: National report on sexual abuse and sexual harassment at Australian universities.* Retrieved from https://www.humanrights.gov.au/our-work/sex-discrimination/publications/change-course-national-report-sexual-assault-and-sexual

Bell, V. (1993). *Interrogating incest. Feminism, foucault and the law.* London: Routledge.

Bondi, L. (2006). Is counselling a feminist practice? *Geo Journal, 65*, 339–348.

Bourke, J. (2012). Sexual violence, bodily pain, and trauma: A history. *Theory, Culture & Society, 29*(3), 25–51. https://doi.org/10.1177/0263276412439406

Breckenridge, J. (1992). An exotic phenomenon? Incest and child rape. In J. Breckenridge & M. Carmody (Eds.), *Crimes of violence. Australian responses to rape and child sexual assault* (pp. 18–37). Allen and Unwin: Sydney.

Breckenridge, J. (1999). Subjugation and silences: The role of the professions in silencing victims of sexual and domestic violence. In J. Breckenridge & L. Laing (Eds.), *Challenging silence. Innovative responses to sexual and domestic violence* (pp. 6–32). St Leonards: Allen & Unwin.

Breckenridge, J., & Laing, L. (Eds.). (1999). *Challenging silence: Innovative responses to sexual and domestic violence.* St Leonards: Allen & Unwin.

Brownmiller, S. (1975). *Against our will: Men, women and rape.* London: Secker, Warburg Simon and Schuster.

Bumiller, K. (2008). *In an abusive state: How neoliberalism appropriated the feminist movement against sexual violence.* Durham, NC: Duke University Press.

Burke, C. (1992). Expert on her own story: Working with women's experiences of incest. In J. Breckenridge & M. Carmody (Eds.), *Crimes of violence. Australian responses to rape and child sexual assault* (pp. 109–120). North Sydney: Allen and Unwin.

Burstow, B. (2005). A critique of posttraumatic stress disorder and the DSM. *Journal of Humanistic Psychology, 45*(4), 429–445.

Carmody, M. (1992). Uniting all women: A historical look at attitudes to rape. In J. Breckenbridge & M. Carmody (Eds.), *Crimes of violence: Australian responses to rape and child sexual assault* (pp. 18–37). Sydney: Allen & Unwin.

Carmody, M. (1995). *Site of struggle: The development of sexual assault services in New South Wales, Australia.* Unpublished doctoral dissertation, University of New South Wales, Australia.

Carmody, M. (2000). Ethical erotics. Reconceptualising anti-rape education. *Sexualities, 8*(4), 465–480.

Case, J. (1992). Meeting others. Groupwork for children who have been sexually abused. In J. Breckenridge & M. Carmody (Eds.), *Crimes of violence. Australian responses to rape and child sexual assault* (pp. 144–150). North Sydney: Allen and Unwin.

Crook, S. (2018). The women's liberation movement, activism and therapy at the grassroots, 1968–1985. *Women's History Review, 27*(7), 1152–1168. https://doi.org/10.1080/09612025.2018.1450611

Cvetkovich, A. (2003). *An archive of feelings: Trauma, sexuality, and lesbian public cultures.* Durham, NC: Duke University Press.

Dworkin, A. (1981). *Pornography: Men possessing women.* London: Women's Press.

Dworkin, A. (1982). *Our blood: Prophecies and discourses on sexual politics.* London: The Women's Press.

Education Centre Against Violence (ECAV). (n.d.-a). *Medical and forensic courses.* Retrieved from http://www.ecav.health.nsw.gov.au/medical-and-forensic-courses/

Education Centre Against Violence (ECAV). (n.d.-b). Courses and forums. Retrieved from http://www.ecav.health.nsw.gov.au/sexual-assault-courses/

Edwards, A. (1987). Male violence in feminist theory: An analysis of the changing conceptions of sex/gender violence and male dominance. In J. Hanmer & M. Maynard (Eds.), *Women, violence and social control* (pp. 13–29). London: Palgrave Macmillan.

Egan, S. (2019). Excavating feminist knowledges and practices in the field of sexual assault service provision: An Australian case study. *Women's Studies International Forum, 74*, 169–178. https://doi.org/10.1016/j.wsif.2019.04.001

Firestone, S. (1970). *The dialectic of sex: The case for feminist revolution*. New York, NY: Morrow.

Franzway, S., Court, D., & Connell, R. W. (1989). *Staking a claim. Feminism, bureaucracy and the state*. North Sydney: Allen and Unwin.

Gavey, N. (2019). *Just sex?: The cultural scaffolding of rape* (2nd ed.). Abingdon & New York, NY: Routledge.

Griffin, S. (1977). Rape. The all American crime. In D. Cahppell, R. Geis, & G. Geis (Eds.), *Forcible rape. The crime, the victim, and the offender* (pp. 47–66). New York, NY: Columbia University Press.

Hall, S. (2004). Foucault and discourse. In C. Seale (Ed.), *Social research methods reader* (pp. 345–349). London: Routledge.

Herman, J. (1997). *Trauma and recovery: The aftermath of violence – from domestic abuse to political terror*. New York, NY: Basic Books.

Hester, M., & Lilley, S.-J. (2017). More than support to court: Rape victims and specialist sexual violence services. *International Review of Victimology, 24*(3), 313–328. https://doi.org/10.1177/0269758017742717

Irwin, J. (2004). *Discounted stories. Lesbians and domestic violence*. Unpublished doctoral dissertation, University of Sydney, Australia.

Jackson, S. (1996). Heterosexuality and feminist theory. In D. Richardson (Ed.), *Theorising heterosexuality* (pp. 21–38). Buckingham: Open University Press.

Jones, H., & Cook, K. (2008). *Rape crisis. Responding to sexual violence*. Dorset: Russell House Publishing.

Kanin, E. J. (1957). Male aggression in dating-courtship relations. *American Journal of Sociology, 63*(2), 197–204. https://doi.org/10.1086/222177

Kanin, E. J. (1969). Selected dyadic aspects of male sex aggression. *The Journal of Sex Research, 5*(1), 12–28. https://doi.org/10.1080/00224496909550593

Kitzinger, C. (1997). Therapy and how it undermines the practice of radical feminism. In D. Bell & R. Klein (Eds.), *Radically speaking. Feminism reclaimed* (pp. 92–101). Melbourne Spinifex Press.

Lamb, S. (1999). Constructing the victim. Popular images and lasting labels. In S. Lamb (Ed.), *New versions of victims: Feminists struggle with the concept* (pp. 108–138). New York, NY & London: New York University Press.

Mann, R., Horsley, P., Barrett, C., & Tinney, J. (2014). *Norma's project: A research study into the sexual assault of older women in Australia*. Retrieved from https://apo.org.au/node/40334

Mardorossian, C. M. (2002). Towards a new feminist theory of rape. *Signs, 27*(3), 743–775.

Marecek, J. (1999). Trauma talk in feminist clinical practice. In S. Lamb (Ed.), *New versions of victims: Feminist struggle with the concept* (pp. 158–182). New York, NY: New York University Press.

Mason, G. (2002). *The spectacle of violence homophobia, gender and knowledge*. London & New York, NY: Routledge.

McCann, I., & Pearlman, L. (1990). *Psychological trauma and the adult survivor: Theory, therapy, and transformation*. New York, NY: Brunner-Routledge.

McKinnon, C. (1982). Feminism, Marxism and the state: An agenda for theory. *Signs. Journal of Women and Culture, 7*(3), 515–544.

McKinnon, C. (1983). Feminism, Marxism, method and the state. Towards feminist jurisprudence. *Signs. Journal of Women in Culture and Society, 8*(4), 635–655.

Millett, K. (1970). *Sexual politics*. Garden City, NY: Doubleday.

NSW Child Sexual Assault Task Force. (1987). *Report of the New South Wales child sexual assault task force to the Hon. Neville Wran, Q.C., M.P, premier of New South Wales, march 1985*. Sydney: New South Wales Government.

NSW Department of Communities and Justice. (n.d.). *Information for victims accessing counselling*. Retrieved from https://www.victimsservices.justice.nsw.gov.au/Pages/vss/vs_counselling/vs_counselling-acs-about.aspx

NSW Government. (2013). Victims Rights and Support Act 2013 (NSW). Retrieved from https://www.legislation.nsw.gov.au/#/view/act/2013/37/full

NSW Health. (2005). *Sexual assault services policy and procedure manual (adult)*. Sydney: NSW Health.

NSW Health. (2020). *Responding to Sexual assault (adult and child) policy and procedures*. Sydney: NSW Health.

NSW Rape Crisis Centre (NSWRCC). (2008). *Annual report 2007/2008 NSW Rape Crisis Centre*. Sydney: NSW Rape Crisis Centre.

Preston, R. (2014). The Australian woman movement, 1880–1914: Sexuality, marriage and consent. *ANU Undergraduate Research Journal, 6*, 15–22.

Rape and Domestic Violence Services Australia (R&DVSA). (2018a). *Submission to the Australian Law Reform Commission review of the family law system issues paper (IP 48)*. Retrieved from www.rape-dvservices.org.au/uploads/main/PDFs/ALRC-Family-Law-Review-RDVSA-Submission-Website.pdf

Rape and Domestic Violence Services Australia (R&DVSA). (2018b). *Submission to the Legal Affairs and Community Safety Committee in relation to the criminal code (Non-consensual sharing of intimate images) amendment bill 2018*. Retrieved from www.rape-dvservices.org.au/uploads/main/PDFs/Image-Based-Abuse-Bill-RDVSA-Submission-Website.pdf

Rape and Domestic Violence Services Australia (R&DVSA). (2019a). *Submission to NSW Law Reform Commission. Consent in relation to sexual offences: Consultation paper 21*. Retrieved from www.rape-dvservices.org.au/uploads/main/PDFs/RDVSA-Consent-Review-CP21-submission-Website.pdf

Rape and Domestic Violence Services Australia (R&DVSA). (2019b). *Submission to Queensland's Legal Affairs and Community Safety Committee's review of the police powers and responsibilities and other legislation amendment bill 2019.* Retrieved from www.rape-dvservices.org.au/uploads/main/PDFs/RDVSA-Submission-to-the-QLD-Police-Powers-Amendment-Bill.pdf

Rape and Domestic Violence Services Australia (R&DVSA). (2019c). *Submission to the NSW Law Reform Commission's review of consent in relation to sexual offences - draft proposals.* Retrieved from www.rape-dvservices.org.au/uploads/main/PDFs/RDVSA-Final-NSWLRC-submission-on-Draft-Proposals.pdf

Rich, A. (1980). Compulsory heterosexuality and lesbian existence *Signs. Journal of Women and Culture, 5*(4), 631–660.

Robinson, A., & Hudson, K. (2011). Different yet complementary: Two approaches to supporting victims of sexual violence in the UK. *Criminology & Criminal Justice, 11*(5), 515–533. https://doi.org/10.1177/1748895811419972

Russell, D. E. H. (1984). *Sexual exploitation: Rape, child sexual abuse, and workplace harassment.* California, CA: Sage.

Sawer, M. (1990). *Sisters in suits. Women and public policy in Australia.* North Sydney: Allen & Unwin.

Stark, E. (2007). *Coercive control: How men entrap women in personal life.* New York, NY: Oxford University Press.

Walby, S. (2011). *The future of feminism.* Cambridge: Polity Press.

Waldby, C., & Women Against Incest (NSW). (1985). *Breaking the silence: A report based upon the findings of the Women Against Incest Phone-in Survey.* Haberfield: Women Against Incest.

Weeks, W. (1993). Women's contribution to community services. In J. Inglis & L. Rogan (Eds.), *Beyond swings and roundabouts* (pp. 67–79). Sydney: Pluto Press.

CHAPTER 4

Sexual Assault as Trauma

> While it is possible to sit back in the academy and deliver a compelling critique of 'real world' practices, there is something naggingly unsatisfying about critiques that demolish practices that attempt to be liberatory on the grounds that they aren't really. It is not that these critiques aren't valuable or essential, even, but they can't be the last word when there are ongoing pragmatic decisions that have to be made about social action. (Gavey, 2003, p. 203)

Introduction

The next two chapters focus on the place of trauma in work against sexual assault. The increasing dominance of psychological trauma as the accepted way of understanding and responding to sexual violence has been a subject of concern in feminist scholarship (Burstow, 2005; Cvetkovich, 2003; Gavey & Schmidt, 2011; Lamb, 1999; Marecek, 1999; Wilkin & Hillock, 2014). Much of the concern focuses on the imposition of the diagnostic category of PTSD and the incursion of medicine and psychiatry into

---

This chapter includes some extracts from an article I published in 2016 in *Feminist Review* (2016). Thanks to SAGE Publications for permission to use extracts from S. Egan (2016), Sexual assault as trauma: A Foucauldian examination of knowledge practices in the field of sexual assault service provision. Feminist Review 112, 95–112.

S. Egan, *Putting Feminism to Work*,
https://doi.org/10.1007/978-3-030-22109-6_4

feminist work that this represents. Framing the ways women endeavour to cope with sexual violence as symptoms or deficits to be treated, it is argued, not only pathologises victims (Burstow, 2005; Lamb, 1999; Marecek, 1999; Wilkin & Hillock, 2014), but also reduces the issue of sexual violence from a moral and political issue to a mental health problem (Lamb, 1999; Mardorossian, 2002; Marecek, 1999).

While there is acknowledgement by some writers that a focus on suffering and psychological harm has played an important role in feminist work against sexual violence—as instrumental in challenging discourses of silence and blame and in public recognition of sexual violence as a serious social issue (e.g. Lamb, 1999; Mardorossian, 2002; O'Dell, 2003; Reavey, 2003; Reavey & Brown, 2007)—there is concern that the increasing dominance of what Marecek (1999) referred to as 'trauma talk' and O'Dell (2003) as the 'harm story' by feminist practitioners both works against traditional feminist principles that promote strength, choice and autonomy and is indicative of a decline in grassroots activism and politics that once characterised the feminist movement.

A particular focus of concern is the way the preoccupation with psychological harm positions women living with the effects of childhood sexual abuse (e.g. Burman, 2003; Egan, 2016; Hunter, 2010; Levett, 2003; Marecek, 1999; Reavey, 2003, 2010; Reavey & Brown, 2007; Worrell, 2003). There is concern about the ways this focus on risk 'often requires that feminist activists get caught up in taxonomies or symptomologies which seek to demonstrate exactly how and why child sexual abuse is harmful' (O'Dell, 2003, p. 144). The recourse to psychological science and the focus on harm, it is argued, results in feminists being drawn into positioning survivors of child sexual abuse in problematic ways and leads to assumptions that the harm story speaks for all survivors (Hunter, 2010; Lamb, 1999; Mardorossian, 2002; Marecek, 1999; Reavey & Brown, 2007).

Despite these concerns there has been little empirical research by feminist scholars that has investigated the place of trauma and psychological harm in the work of sexual assault services or feminist practitioners. Research to date has provided insights into the uptake of the sexual assault as trauma narrative by community members (Gavey & Schmidt, 2011), by adults survivors of child sexual abuse (Hunter, 2010; O'Dell, 2003; Reavey, 2003; Worrell, 2003) and by a range of professionals (such as mental health, medical, legal professionals as well as therapists) who work with survivors (Marecek, 1999; O'Dell, 2003; Reavey, 2003). Of the later,

Marecek's (1999) which I outlined in Chapter 2, is the sole study to explicitly focus on feminist practitioners.

Gavey and Schmidt (2011) set out to explore everyday understandings of rape and the impact of rape using a focus groups ($n = 29$) made up of community members in New Zealand.

However, they found, that the only understanding of rape present came via a discourse of trauma which they defined as the view that rape is an inherently traumatic experience, that the nature of trauma is psychological and, because of this, rape affects all aspects of a person's life. Further rape was understood as an experience that is more traumatic than other types of traumatic events and, because of this, as having a lifelong legacy. Women who don't acknowledge harm were seen by some participants as being in denial with recovery understood as something that would have to be actively pursued by the victim and would require the support of others, most usually a professional. Similarly, Worrell (2003), in research based on a facilitated self-help group for women sexually abused as children, found that most discussions focused on the long-term harms of the abuse (emotional, psychological and physical), although Worrell does note that participants also emphasised their strength in surviving.

Conversely, Hunter's (2010), research which explored the narratives people construct about their experiences of childhood sexual abuse, found that a narrative of ongoing harm and suffering was just one of four distinctive narratives amongst survivors who had experienced abuse across different social and historical contexts in which understandings of and interventions in relation to child sexual abuse were markedly different compared to today. Based on interviews with 22 Australian women and men of different ages and social backgrounds Hunter (2010) identified the first narrative as one of transcendence where while the person had experienced significant harm was unwilling to talk about this publicly because they did not want to be identified as either victim or survivor and thus have their identity linked to a particular childhood experience/s. Second, the narrative of ongoing harm and suffering where the individual's experiences of abuse and their identity as a survivor did play a central role in their current life. Third, a narrative of transformation in which the person had used their experiences of abuse to help or protect others, and finally a narrative of silence where the person felt they had not been affected by the abuse and did not want to talk to others about it. Significantly the latter group were aware that it was no longer socially acceptable to say that one had not been traumatised or negatively affected and reported that the increased media discussion of the impacts of child sexual assault had resulted in them feeling some pressure that they should 'tell their story'. Indeed, some had begun to question their stance and wonder if there were connections between their abuse and adult difficulties such as problems in their intimate lives (Hunter, 2010, p. 182).

Reavey (2003) explored narratives about the relationships between women survivor's past and present as they appear in therapeutic, self-help and survivor accounts, with focus on how women's sexuality is viewed in relation to past abuse. Based on interviews with ten professionals (i.e. psychologists, psychiatrists, counsellors) in UK public and private sector positions who had worked with adults sexually abused in childhood, ten survivors of childhood sexual abuse and four popular self-help texts, she found that the cause of difficulties in adult sexual relationships were invariably attributed to their childhood sexual abuse. She argues that this narrow psychological focus elides the social and cultural context through which gendered sexual relationships are enacted, instead producing difficulties encountered as symptoms or effects of prior abuse.

O'Dell (2003) explored how the harm of child sexual abuse was understood in relation to the concept of childhood development, using data from interviews with professionals (from medical, legal, social work and therapist backgrounds) who worked with adults or children who had a history of child sexual abuse and women and men who identified themselves as survivors of child sexual abuse. She found that the 'harm story' positioned adults who were subject to sexual victimisation in childhood as qualitatively different from non-abused others. Understood through the psychological lens of childhood development, the harm of child sexual assault is understood as a series of ongoing problems which can be reactivated by adult life events and developmental stages. For example, entering an adult sexual relationship or having a child may trigger distressing memories or feelings associated with the abuse.

In a related study Warner (2003) examined how women who have been sexually abused are spoken about and understood in secure mental hospitals. Her study consisted of data collected from patients and professionals (drawn from all ranks within the hospitals, including psychiatrists, occupational therapists, social workers, pharmacists) from two British maximum-security mental hospitals. Warner focuses on the frequency with which the women were diagnosed with borderline personality disorder (BDP) and argues that this diagnosis obscures the social causes of women misery. In addition, she found that even where childhood sexual abuse was accorded a role in the development of mental illness, it was used to signal pathology.

For example, she highlights instances where the professionals had used the patient's history of child sexual abuse to support a diagnosis of BPD on the basis that child sexual abuse has an adverse effect on personality development.

Finally, Marecek (1999), who set out to investigate how feminist therapists use feminism in their work, found instead that that 'trauma talk' dominated the interviews she and her master's degree students conducted with 40 feminist therapists in one US state. Although participants were employed in a variety of contexts—rather than specially as sexual assault counsellors, they nevertheless typically framed the current difficulties their clients brought to therapy as the result of childhood abuse, which, as I laid out in Chapter 2, they understood using the concept of PTSD.

Collectively, these studies draw attention to the propensity for the trauma narrative to position survivors as irremediably harmed if not damaged by their abusive experiences and highlight the respective researchers concerns about both the lack of agency afforded to victims through the imposition of medicalised understandings of sexual abuse and the concomitant decline in attention to the social and political context that enables sexual violence.

Through these next two chapters, I use the empirical work I conducted in the field of NSW sexual assault service provision to enter into a dialogue with this scholarship and provide an alternative perspective on the uptake of trauma in feminist work, as well as an insight into what this looks like in an applied field of practice. To the practitioners who worked with victims and survivors on a daily basis, trauma not only 'made sense', it was considered an integral part of their feminist practice. In seeking to understand how trauma was put to work, I drew on Foucault's (1998) methodological concept of the polyvalence of discourse that highlights the variability within a single discourse, depending on how it is deployed. The same discourse can have multiple, even opposing, effects, depending on who is speaking and acting; the institution from which they speak and act; and their position and relative power within that institutional location. Consequently, Foucault (1998) stresses it is not possible to divide discourses into acceptable or excluded, good or bad, just or unjust. Indeed, he argues that a discourse is never just an instrument or effect of power but has the potential to function as a form of resistance, 'the starting point for an opposing strategy' (p. 101). For the purposes of my research, this meant I was able to move away from a position where recourse to diagnostic categories such as PTSD or complex PTSD (c-PTSD) is viewed as implicitly negative or as immediate evidence of a decline in feminism.

Instead, my aim was to elicit and analyse data in a way that would help me understand how these concepts were understood and put to work by sexual assault practitioners, rather than the preoccupation with their status as psychiatric or medical concepts. This enabled me to understand the relationship between the contemporary understanding of sexual assault as an ontological assault, as an assault on the self, and the deployment of trauma. The self in contemporary Western societies is understood through a psychological framework of ideas and concepts, and the harm done to the self by sexual assault is made visible through the concept of psychological trauma. Although this concept illuminates the harm experienced by all victims of sexual assault, it is most carefully articulated and most crucial to the formation of a particular type of victim, the 'adult survivor' of childhood sexual abuse.

Sexual Assault as an Assault on the Self

Foucault (1988), in arguing that sexuality should not be subject to repressive power, proposed that rape be prosecuted not as a sexual crime but as a physical assault, making the provocative statement that 'there is no difference, in principle, between sticking one's fist into someone's face or one's penis into their sex' (p. 200). The usefulness of this stark imagery is that it so vividly illuminates the inadequacy of this representation in capturing contemporary understandings and experiences of sexual violence. As Bourke (2009) points out, it is not possible given current Western notions of sexuality to claim the genitals have the same significance as a fist.

Sexual assault is much more than a physical assault. Across the practitioner interview texts, sexual violence was consistently represented as a qualitatively different type of abuse, one that had particularly serious and ongoing effects. These effects appear linked to a conceptual understanding of sexual assault as an assault on the victim's identity, on her sense of self. The following extracts, selected from the interview texts, are typical of how practitioners described the effects of sexual assault on victims. Implicitly, the types of effects represented communicate something about the concept of sexual assault, about 'what sexual assault is'. The first excerpt is illustrative of sexual assault's positioning as a violation of the self:

> I think it affects every part of their life really. I mean, we talked about it and said it was a violation and it's a violation of every part of their being, you

know. I think there is no other crime that really affects a person on every level—you know, it affects physically, mentally, emotionally, spiritually. (Interview Text No. 7)

Sexual assault is a 'violation' that affects the victim on 'every level' of their being.

Again, the next excerpt represents sexual assault as an assault on the victim's personhood, as an assault on the self:

> I think that sexual violence is something that really—it's such an assault on yourself. I mean, it's a bodily assault but, I mean, when you see how much it affects people's sense of who they are and where they are in the world and their safety in the world and see how that affects how they relate to their families and what it does to their relationships and then you see how that affects parenting and then later on down the line when people haven't had that sort of—that sense of how to protect themselves from danger and sort of the increased vulnerability that comes with being victimised. And how that then carries on. (Interview Text No. 19)

Sexual assault is 'a bodily assault', but it is much more than that: It is an assault on the self. Although the corporeality of sexual assault is referenced, the subsequent list of effects is psychological and relational. It affects victims' relationships with their families, with themselves, their 'sense of who they are' and their place 'in the world'. The effect on the victim's subsequent safety appears positioned as a psychological effect. There is something about the experience of sexual assault that leaves the victim 'vulnerable' and unable to 'protect themselves from danger' in the future. Similarly, the effect on the victim's capacity to parent appears positioned as a long- term psychological effect. It is something that happens 'down the line'. In this excerpt, the practitioner has built a relationship between the concept of sexual assault as an assault on the self and a series of psychological and relational effects that appear as consequences of the injury to the self. The next excerpt, presented in two parts, begins with the effects of sexual assault on the victim's identity, on their sense of self:

I guess the major effects are about how people see themselves and how they value themselves. I guess that identity—so it affects self-esteem, it affects confidence, it affects people's ability to trust that the world, as we know it, is a safe place that they can live in. (Interview Text. No. 28)

The next part continues to lay out the ways sexual assault affects the victim's views of and experiences in the 'world':

> So people's worldviews, I often talk about how assault will impact and change a person's worldview and trying to assist people to see that, that world you can come back to what it was prior to the assault. Look it affects people's livelihoods, it affects their relationships with other people, how they communicate, it affects how people can connect even with themselves and others—sexual assault can often result in people having a disconnection from their bodies, not being able to see their bodies as a safe place to be in. It can result in being disconnected from other people as well because they don't see themselves as the same. They see themselves as being damaged and different. (Interview Text No. 28)

One recurring theme in this representation is disconnection. Sexual assault affects victims' capacity to connect with themselves, with their bodies and with other people. The disconnection appears related to the ways the experience of sexual assault changes victims' sense of safety—in the world and in their bodies—and changes how they see themselves. They see themselves as 'damaged' and as 'different' to other people.

The interview text excerpts above all contain lists of consequences, and these lists work to produce sexual violence as a specific type of seriously harmful event. This technique is consistent across the library of documents (service brochures, information booklets, policy manuals) where lists of harms are used to underline the consequences of sexual assault. However, the interview texts make explicit what remains implicit in other documents: that sexual assault is an ontological assault, an assault on the self. The broader effects of sexual assault are consequences of the ontological changes to the victim. Because of the injury to the self caused by sexual assault, victims have trouble with their families, in relationships, in communicating with others, in feeling safe, in keeping themselves safe and in caring for their children. This representation of 'what sexual assault is' relies upon a particular understanding of personhood. As Rose (1996) points out, the contemporary Western conception of the person is of an individualised and internalised self, stable across time and context. In Western societies, the self 'is construed as a naturally unique and discrete entity, the boundaries of the body enclosing, as if by definition, an inner life of the psyche, in which are inscribed the experiences of an individual biography' (Rose, 1996, p. 103). Sexual assault does involve bodies—the body of the victim and the body of the perpetrator—but it is much more than an assault on the body. The significance of the sexed parts of the body in contemporary understandings of sexuality and the centrality of sexuality to identity means sexual violence is an assault on the self: a physical violation *and* a violation of the inner psyche. It is within this contemporary understanding of personhood that sexual abuse is produced as a serious violation of the person. Rose (1996, p. 103) argues that Western societies are unusual in their understanding of the self as the origin point of actions and decisions, the place in which beliefs and desires are located. He points out that in these societies, psychology was born as a scientific discipline, based on knowledge of the self, with a particular truth about selves and practices for acting upon them. In the practitioner interview texts, the harm of sexual violence becomes visible using the language of psychological trauma.

Trauma as Symptomatic of an Assault on the Self

Trauma emerged as a dominant concept, with the term and its variants circulating through the practitioner interview texts and appearing as trauma, sexual abuse trauma, complex trauma, post-traumatic stress and vicarious trauma. Often, the term was used factually without explanation or elaboration. Victims of sexual assault were described as 'very, very traumatised' and their reactions as 'about trauma—all the reactions to trauma'. Sexual assault was discussed as affecting people 'more than other forms of trauma'. 'Untreated trauma' was often the core issue identified by practitioners as underlying other problems, drug and alcohol problems or mental illness. Sexual assault practitioners often experienced 'vicarious trauma', and practitioners new to the field 'have to know about trauma' in order to work effectively with victims of sexual assault. The frequency with which 'trauma' appeared in the texts and the factual manner in which it was used suggests a naturalised relationship had been established between sexual assault and trauma. As Foucault (1972, p. 57) points out, naturalised relationships between concepts can be formed either explicitly or implicitly, through sophisticated arguments or through 'ordinary statements'. Their existence may be confirmed formally through science or through recourse to tradition, authority or 'mere repetition' (p. 57). Indeed, as discussed in the previous chapter, it is often the lack of explanation, the common-sense everyday way an idea, theory or concept comes to be used that indicates its transition to an uncontested 'truth' (Hall, 2004, p. 78). If sexual assault *is* about gender, power and violence, it *is* also about trauma.

Although often unexplained, there are examples through the interview texts where practitioners explained the relationship between trauma and sexual assault. In these explanations, the violation of the self becomes visible as the concept underpinning the relationship between sexual assault and psychological trauma. The following excerpt is a typical representation:

> I suppose today when I'm using the word trauma, I'm thinking of the psychological impacts of trauma. And I think I'm talking about where there's, sort of, in that traditional sense of a major violation or shock to the person. So something where they've felt like that—the integrity to self is really violated and that's the clinical way of sort of saying it. But any—in terms of sexual assault, I think any sexual assault sort of fits that description. It is a major violation of your own body or mind and it's, for us, it's the sexual nature in some way, to some degree. (Interview Text No. 23)

Trauma, 'psychological' trauma, happens when the 'self' has been 'really violated', and all forms of sexual assault fit that description. In the first part of the excerpt, the practitioner implies there are other types of experiences that cause 'major violation or shock'. However, in the last sentence, there is a suggestion of sexual assault as a particularly serious violation. It is a violation of the 'body or mind', but it is also 'the sexual nature' that appears to constitute sexual assault as a particular type of trauma and violation.

The interview texts contain a common pattern of psychological and emotional effects presented as aggregations and symptoms including nightmares, fear of going out, anxiety, difficulty in concentrating and fears of victims that they are going mad. These types of 'symptoms' are routinely anchored using the concept of trauma and variously described as the 'effects of trauma', 'PTSD symptoms' and 'post-traumatic stress'.

The following excerpts illustrate the repetition with which trauma symptoms are represented as effects of sexual victimisation. The first excerpt begins by citing the frequency with which victims present with symptoms of PTSD as evidence that sexual assault is a form of trauma:

> The people that we see experience most of the post-traumatic stress symptoms—that's my evidence that sexual violence is trauma. You know, they

> have intrusion; they normally have flashbacks, nightmares, hyper-vigilance, insomnia, depression, anxiety—which I kind of see as falling into the DSM [*Diagnostic and Statistical Manual of Mental Disorders*] definition of trauma, post-traumatic stress. So I would say that everyone that I would see would have some symptomology of trauma. (Interview Text No. 7)

The following excerpt repeats a number of the trauma symptoms cited in the previous excerpt, including hyper-vigilance, nightmares and flashbacks:

> Oh, they become hyper-vigilant, the classic symptoms of post-traumatic stress disorder—startled response, hyper-vigilant, some physiological disorders, eating or not eating, not sleeping, nightmares, flashbacks. (Interview Text No. 2)

In the next excerpt, the practitioner has commented that victims describe their reactions to sexual assault as feeling as if they are 'going crazy'. Asked to explain this type of reaction, the practitioner says the 'crazy' feeling is about the victim having dreams.

> Dreams and the thoughts—not being able to concentrate, leaving things—put something down, can't find it. It's like overload of the brain. So it's about trauma—all the reactions to trauma. (Interview Text No. 10)

The dreams, thoughts, lack of concentration, the forgetfulness are all 'reactions to trauma'. Much of the terminology present in these excerpts—'intrusion', 'nightmares', 'flashbacks', 'hyper-vigilance', 'physiological disorders'—is also used to define the diagnostic criteria for PTSD.

PTSD was formally recognised in 1980 when it was included in the third edition of the DSM, the official nosology of the American Psychiatric Association (Young, 1995, p. 7). In the aftermath of the Vietnam war, veterans' groups in the United States played a significant role in advocating for recognition of what had been considered a character weakness (war neurosis) as a legitimate disorder caused by the horrors they had experienced and witnessed during the war.

Indeed, the fundamental impetus in the creation of a diagnostic manual was to move psychiatry away from psychoanalytic thinking that attributes mental illness to unseen processes originating in the individual psyche. Spitzer, the architect of the wide-reaching changes brought about by DSM-III, aimed to devise a classificatory system that, like medicine, would be based on empirical observation and measurement and allow researchers and clinicians across theoretical perspectives to communicate about the same set of disorders (Young, 1995).

Like most diagnostic categories, PTSD has undergone a number of iterations, with changes in the definition of what constitutes a traumatic event and in symptomology (Young, 1995). For example, changes between the previous manual (DSM-IV) and current (DSM-5) include specific naming of sexual violence in the definition of what constitutes a traumatic event and removal of the requirement that the person react to that event in a particular way (fear, horror) as part of this definition.[1] Without negating these changes, the core features of PTSD as described by Herman (1992b) in *Trauma and Recovery* and as used in applied, non-psychiatric settings remain consistent. Victims of PTSD typically experience heightened levels of physiological arousal (e.g. startling easily, problems with sleep) and tend to cycle between being flooded with distressing memories of the traumatic experience and trying to avoid anything that reminds them of the experience and/or feeling emotionally numb and distant from self and others.

To provide a more rounded description, DSM-5 describes PTSD as follows: The person has been exposed to actual or threatened death, serious injury or sexual violence. This person may be the victim of this event or events, have witnessed the event as it happened or be impacted either because they are a close friend or relative of the victim[2] or a professional exposed firsthand to aversive details of the events (e.g. police officer, medical practitioner, counsellor). The symptoms of PTSD are divided into four criteria—intrusive, avoidance, alternations in arousal and reactivity

[1] In addition, PTSD is now categorised under the new category of Trauma and Stressor-Related Disorders rather than under Anxiety Disorders, as it had in previous versions of the manual. This change is reported to have occurred to reflect that people with PTSD respond with a range of emotions outside the fear/anxiety constellation (Pai, Suris, & North, 2017). The emotional reactions to the traumatic event are now captured in an additional set of symptoms that focus on emotional and cognitive changes and have been extended to include feelings such as guilt and shame that are more often the response of sexual assault victims—for example, victims who know the person who abused them may not necessarily react with fear or horror. In addition, a specific group of criteria has been added for children aged six years and younger to reflect their developmental stage. For example, with young children, the persistent remembering might be in the form of play and may not necessarily cause the child overt distress.

[2] In relation to friends or relatives, the actual or threatened death is limited to violent or unexpected deaths (American Psychiatric Association, 2013).

and negative alterations in cognition and mood (American Psychiatric Association, 2013) and can be summarised as follows:

1. **Intrusive**. The traumatic event or events are persistently re-experienced—for example, through nightmares, upsetting or involuntary and unwanted memories or dissociative reactions such as flashbacks in which the person feels and reacts as if the traumatic event is reoccurring; significant and prolonged psychological distress and/or marked physiological reactivity after exposure to the traumatic reminders.
2. **Avoidance**. The individual persistently avoids stimuli associated with the event or events—for example, avoids distressing memories, thoughts or feelings about the traumatic event/s and/or avoids external reminders (people, places, situations) that arouse the former.
3. **Alterations in arousal and reactivity**. Significant arousal or reactivity that begins or worsens after the event/s and that includes two or more of the following symptoms: sleep disturbance, exaggerated startle response, hyper-arousal, poor concentration, irritable and angry outbursts, reckless or self-destructive behaviours.
4. **Negative alterations in cognition and mood** beginning or worsening after the traumatic event/s. Specific symptoms include persistent negative emotional state (i.e. fear, horror, guilt, shame, anger) and/or inability to experience positive emotions. The person may show a marked disinterest in participating in significant activities and/or feel detached or estranged from others. They may experience a distorted sense of blame of self or others or an inability to remember an important part of the event/s.[3]

Thus, sexual assault, as an experience that produces symptoms of trauma (PTSD), is established as a serious and harmful event. Moreover, establishing a relationship between sexual assault and PTSD also establishes a relationship between sexual assault and other serious events such as witnessing a murder, physical assault and other socially recognised

[3] The addition of three new symptoms—persistent negative emotional states, reckless or self-destructive behaviour and 'distorted' cognitions about the trauma that lead to self-blame or blaming others—has been critiqued, including by some within the psychiatric community, as both pathologising and introducing characteristics of personality disorders into the PTSD diagnosis (Pai et al., 2017).

experiences of violence and harm. The reactions of the sexual assault victim, the physiological, psychological, emotional and behavioural reactions, are not symptoms of 'craziness' but the expected and accepted (or medically sanctioned) reactions to a serious and harmful event (Herman, 1997).

In most interview texts, practitioners carefully avoided using the term 'disorder', instead favouring the descriptor 'post-traumatic stress' or the abbreviation 'PTSD', as exemplified by the previous excerpts. Others distinguished between PTSD as a 'clinical' or diagnostic term and their own more general use as a descriptor of reactions to trauma. However, regardless of the specific term used, PTSD was employed consistently to position victims' reactions as 'normal' reactions to a serious event. PTSD therefore functions as an important tool of legitimation, both of the serious nature of sexual assault and of the psychological injury—the injury to the psyche—sustained by the victim (Herman, 1997).

This naturalisation of trauma, the way terms like PTSD and 'traumatised' are used to convey the violation to the self that lies at the heart of the contemporary experience of sexual violence, suggests that trauma in this context functions as a concept that conveys empathy and understanding rather than as a diagnostic tool that is imposed or used to identify deficits. Fassin and Rechtman (2009), in *The Empire of Trauma: An Inquiry into the Condition of Victimhood*, argue that trauma has become part of our moral economy, a 'floating signifier' that expresses legitimacy and empathy towards victims and signals 'complaints as justified and causes as just' (p. 277). Its use as a diagnostic category, they suggest, at most reinforces this legitimacy. The idea that tragic and painful events, whether individually or collectively experienced, leave marks in the mind, which are then seen as 'scars by analogy to those left on the body' (p. 4), is accepted within contemporary society. It indicates how violence and misfortune are understood in contemporary Western societies 'as phenomena that leave traces of the past in the present, and that may even require immediate treatment to ensure they do not' (p. 4). The language of trauma, which fewer than 30 years ago was rarely invoked outside 'the closed circles of psychiatry and psychology' (p. 284), has become part of everyday usage.

Trauma and the 'Adult Survivor'

The concept of trauma coalesces most densely in the interview texts where the focus is adult survivors of childhood sexual abuse, routinely referred to by the shorthand term 'adult survivors'. The adult survivor appears an unstable subject through the interview texts. Adult survivors are described as living with multiple psychological and emotional problems as a consequence of childhood abuse, including 'constant nightmares, drug abuse, on pills, in and out of hospital, suicidal, self-harm' (Interview Text No. 2). They appear to struggle in their adult social and intimate relationships, often experiencing 'issues around intimacy', with feeling a 'sense of isolation' from others that can be compounded by difficulties in 'communicating in a social setting' (Interview Text No. 11). Their abusive childhood experiences have often left adult survivors 'vulnerable to ongoing abuse' (Interview Text No. 17), and as a population group, they experience a high rate of sexual 're-victimisation' in adulthood (Interview Text No. 20). Thus, the adult survivor was positioned across the texts as the category of victim for whom sexual victimisation had the most serious and ongoing consequences.

This ongoing harm was encapsulated through the concept of 'complex trauma'. While all victims of sexual assault were positioned as 'traumatised', the 'complexity' of the trauma experienced distinguished adult survivors from other victims—for example, adult victims of recent rape. Although sharing a 'familial' resemblance to PTSD, 'complex trauma' is a distinctive type of trauma and, as implied by the term, is understood as a particularly injurious form of trauma, one that has multiple, complicated and long-term effects. The following excerpts are illustrative of how the complexity of trauma experienced by adult survivors of child sexual assault is represented across the interview texts. The excerpt begins by reference to 'two different' populations of victims:

> I was talking about the two different populations and the impacts. So I think the impacts for a person who has a good enough childhood, grown up and then experienced adulthood sexual assault, I think that all of the symptoms [PTSD] that we've talked about can be experienced by that group of people. The other group of people are people who experienced traumas including sexual assault trauma during childhood and I think of people in that situation as people who have a complexity of trauma. And in that, the trauma that they experienced during childhood interrupted development at crucial stages. And that often what I see happening is that people who experienced child sexual assault, adult survivors of childhood sexual assault, can present with a combination of symptoms that is rarely seen in the adult population of people that had a good enough childhood and the trauma during adulthood. (Interview Text No. 3)

The core differences between the 'populations' appear related to the concept of a 'good enough childhood'. Adult victims who have had a 'good enough' childhood experience the simpler form of trauma, PTSD. Adult victims of childhood trauma, which includes 'sexual assault trauma', experience a more complex form of trauma and experience symptoms 'rarely seen' in the other 'population'. The attribution for the trauma's complexity is represented as two-tiered: the 'sexual trauma' experienced and the effect of that experience on childhood development. In the second part of the excerpt, the practitioner lays out the sorts of 'difficulties' that come with complex trauma:

> And I think that those difficulties show up often in terms of interpersonal and intrapersonal skills. So the abilities to self-regulate. The ability to have a reference point for what crisis isn't. And I guess a whole bunch of things around that but I think adult survivors of childhood sexual assault can, don't always, but can present with a more complex range of symptoms. An additional layer, I suppose, for this population which is that also the development of key skills was not developed. So the interpersonal effectiveness, the distress toleration, the emotion regulation—those sorts of intrapersonal skills and interpersonal skills. (Interview Text No. 3)

Adult survivors can, although it is stressed do not always, 'present with a more complex range of symptoms' than adult rape victims. These symptoms, as I go on to discuss in the next section, are the difficulty in regulating emotions and tolerating distress and the problems experienced in interpersonal relationships associated with c-PTSD (Burke, Mulder, Gravina, Walker, & Dombrowski, 2014; Cloitre et al., 2011; Herman, 2012). The point I want to highlight now is the place of childhood abuse and childhood development in the aetiology of these more complex effects. As the practitioner above points out towards the end of the first excerpt, the difference with complex trauma is 'that the trauma that they experienced during childhood interrupted development at crucial stages' (Interview Text No. 3). Yet child victims, as opposed to adults who had been victims of sexual abuse in childhood, appeared infrequently in the interview discussions of 'complex trauma' or of PTSD, although at times they were described using the generic descriptor 'traumatised'.

In the next excerpt, the practitioner lays out the differences she had found between working with child victims and with adult survivors of child sexual assault. In particular, she highlights the speed with which children move through the counselling process. Importantly, she also draws attention to the factors that mean child victims and adult survivors, while both sexually victimised during childhood, can experience different sets of consequences and become positioned as essentially different 'types' of victims:

> I think children developmentally also move—just children move through the process faster and they tend to do bits and pieces of the process, like they might come to counselling for a short period of time but then they sort of go and do their life or they come back when Court's going on. It's a really—and generally speaking, the fact that a child is engaged in the counselling process, there's a supportive—generally there's a supportive carer or parent which is the key—I mean, at the end of the day the key issue is being believed and safety and the abuse stopping and having safe relationships. So for a lot of children, counselling is resourcing, hopefully icing on the cake. Yes, they're very traumatised but you've got a supportive carer and intervening at a much earlier age and they really run with it. I found starting to work with adults, how much it really showed me about sort of even—I needed to learn so much more about the impact on relationships—like how much more time I needed to address issues that would arise in the therapeutic relationship, if that makes sense? (Interview Text No. 17)

If a child victim is in counselling, it means the abuse has stopped. It means that they are safe. It means that they have had the reparative experience of having their account believed, and it means they have a supportive parent or carer. As the practitioner goes on to explain, for many children in such circumstances, the 'interventions' have happened earlier, while they are still young. In this type of scenario, counselling is 'icing on the cake' for a lot of children.

This suggests that the complexity of the consequences for 'adult survivors' is not solely about disrupted development but also about not being believed as children, of not having supportive parents or access to counselling or other types of ameliorative interventions. This suggests sexual victimisation in childhood does not automatically lead to problems in adult functioning. The difference between the child victim and the 'adult survivor' is represented in this excerpt and across the interview texts as a function of the time gap between the abuse and the intervention, together with a number of absences—for example, of a supportive parent or of the experience of being believed when they disclosed the abuse.

The relationship between abusive childhood experiences and adult problems does lie, however, at the heart of 'complex trauma'. As I set out through the remainder of the chapter, the nature of the relationship between past abuse and problems in adulthood hinge on three sets of often-unarticulated ideas: first, a specific set of ideas about childhood development; second, a particular understanding of how traumatic experiences interrupt and affect that development; and third, the process by which this interruption produces a recognisable set of symptoms or effects in the now-adult subject.

Complex Trauma

Unlike PTSD, complex trauma has not been included in the DSM, although attempts were made for both DSM-IV and DSM-5[4] (e.g. Resick et al., 2012; Roth, Newman, Pelcovitz, van der Kolk, & Mandel, 1997; van der Kolk, Roth, Pelcovitz, Sunday, & Spinazzola, 2005). However, it is typically referred to both by trauma researchers (e.g. Cloitre, Garvert, Brewin, Bryant, & Maercker, 2013; Courtois & Ford, 2009; Karatzias & Cloitre, 2019) and in practice publications referenced and used in NSW and wider Australian sexual assault service sectors as a clinically recognised condition (e.g. Burke et al., 2014; Davidson, 2007; Kezelman & Stavropolous, 2018, 2019). The increasing recognition and acceptance of the concept of complex trauma in the field of sexual assault service provision is reflected in the provision of specific training workshops on understanding and responding to complex trauma by organisations such as the Education Centre Against Violence (ECAV) and Rape and Domestic Violence Services Australia (R&DVSA) as well as specific reference to complex trauma in the newly released NSW Health policy and practice guidelines *Responding to Sexual Assault (Adult and Child) Policy and*

[4]Complex PTSD has recently been included in the latest version of the World Health Organization's (WHO's) International Classification of Diseases (ICD, 2018), replacing the personality disorder enduring personality changes after catastrophic events (EPCACE; Karatzias & Levendosky, 2019). However, the DSM is the most widely recognised and used diagnostic system in Australia (Price-Robertson, 2018). In addition, it has been pointed out that some of the additional symptoms included in DSM-5 resemble the cluster of symptoms typically associated with c-PTSD. An example is the inclusion of a dissociative PTSD subtype in which the person experiences a sense of depersonalisation—feeling detached from their body, mind or sensations and/or derealisation, which refers to a feeling of being detached or cut off from their surroundings (Giourou et al., 2018).

Procedures (2020).[5] Typically, PTSD is understood as inadequate in capturing the complicated and interrelated effects of prolonged abuse, particularly chronic abuse in childhood. Consequently, complex trauma or c-PTSD includes the core effects associated with PTSD (the re-experiencing, avoidance, numbing and hyper-arousal) as well as more diffuse difficulties across three additional domains: problems in regulating emotions, pronounced difficulties in forming and maintaining relationships and a negative belief system about oneself, for example, that results in deep-seated feelings of worthlessness and shame (Cloitre et al., 2011; Giourou et al., 2018; Karatzias & Levendosky, 2019). The types of difficulties often described in relation to complex trauma include the types of difficulties often described in relation to complex trauma, including self-harm, suicidality, ongoing difficulties in interpersonal relationships, periods of dissociation, pervasive feelings of shame and re-victimisation in adulthood.

Complex Trauma, Child Sexual Abuse and the Mental Health System

The term 'complex PTSD' was first coined by Judith Herman (1992a), the US feminist psychiatrist whose text *Trauma and Recovery: From Domestic Abuse to Political Terror* (1992b) was frequently referred to in the interview texts as 'the bible'. Herman explicitly situated herself and her work as feminist, and the key argument she pursued through *Trauma and Recovery* was that social and political recognition of victims of 'trauma' (whether war veterans or victims of sexual abuse) occurs only in the context of a strong political movement.

[5] Examples of the types of training workshops include a one-day Overview of Dialectical Behaviour Therapy (DBT) in Responding to People with Complex Trauma available through ECAV (2019) and a two-day Understanding and Responding to Complex Trauma provided by R&DVSA (2019). In addition Australia's National Research Organisation for Women's Safety (ANROWS) recently provided funding for research focusing on improving service responses to women with experiences of complex trauma—Salter, M., Conroy, E., Dragiewicz, M., Burke, J., Ussher, J., Middleton, W., Vilenica, S., Martin Monzon, B., & Noack-Lundberg, K. (2020). 'A deep wound under my heart': Constructions of complex trauma and implications for women's wellbeing and safety from violence (Research report, 12/2020). Sydney, Australia: ANROWS.

http://www.nasasv.org.au/index.htm.

In *Trauma and Recovery*, Herman (1992b) argues that the experience and effects of sexual and domestic violence, like the experience and effects of war, should be understood as trauma specifically (PTSD), which had been accepted as a formal diagnosis in DSM-III in 1980 (Young, 1995, p. 7). However, a primary focus of this text proposes the necessity for an additional diagnostic category of c-PTSD. Herman (1992) argues that PTSD does not capture the complex symptoms of victims who have experienced prolonged, repeated abuse. Her proposal focuses most specifically on the consequences of abuse experienced in childhood, particularly child sexual abuse, which she argues are more pervasive and insidious because they interrupt the development of the child's psychological, emotional and cognitive capacities. As a result, adult victims of childhood sexual abuse often experience problems whose aetiology can be traced to untreated early childhood trauma, including difficulties in their adulthood relationships, with identity formation and self-perception, and vulnerability to further harm to themselves and from others, including adult sexual victimisation.

Further, Herman (1992b) proposes c-PTSD as an alternative to the pejorative diagnosis of BPD.[6] Citing her own and others' research on the rates of childhood abuse in the histories of these patients, Herman proposes their often-problematic symptoms, similar to those proposed as criteria for c-PTSD, are better understood within the framework of c-PTSD as the effects of childhood abuse. Herman (1992b) is critical of the treatment that survivors of child abuse receive in mental health systems and considers that, by treating symptoms as causes, professionals working in these systems continue the culture of blaming the victim by focusing on the victim's inherent character as the source of the problem.[7] More recently, some trauma theorists, such as John Briere and colleagues (e.g. Briere, 2002; Briere & Jordan, 2009; Briere, Kaltman, & Green, 2008), have moved beyond personality disorders to conceptualise other mental illnesses such as depression, anxiety and schizophrenia as effects of childhood abuse.

[6] The psychoanalyst Adolph Stern first used the term 'borderline group' in 1938 to describe a condition that fell between psychotic and neurotic disorders (Kulkarni, 2017), although BPD was not recognised as a diagnosable personality disorder until 1980 (Shaw & Proctor, 2005).

[7] Since proposing c-PTSD as a diagnostic category in 1992, Herman has remained critical of its lack of inclusion in the DSM. See, for example, her response to Resick et al. (2012) about the decision not to include c-PTSD in DSM- 5 (Herman, 2012).

Following Herman, the sexual assault practitioners I interviewed viewed BPD as the epitome of the poor treatment of victims of childhood sexual abuse, the most pronounced example of how the 'medical model' forecloses the individual, and their perceived deficits, as the source of the problem. Sexual assault practitioners represented 'complex trauma' as a mechanism that enabled them to challenge the pathologisation of 'adult survivors', particularly within the mental health system. In the following excerpt, a practitioner with many years' experience working in the sexual assault services sector reflects on the role trauma came to play when it began to emerge in these services:

> And very much sort of challenging perhaps the medical mainstream sort of health models, and very much learning to understand sexual assault in the context of trauma and psychological trauma rather than pathologising and totalising women and children's experiences as being somehow mental health deficits. So really trying to take the—I think what particularly [names of services] were doing were taking the impacts and effects and really challenging that they weren't—that they were very normal, expected effects of terrible trauma and were not mental health dysfunction. As what was a lot in the medical literature. (Interview Text No. 17)

This type of positioning runs through the interview texts. Rather than a form of medical or medicalised knowledge, the concept of psychological trauma is understood as a concept that can and has been used to challenge the 'medical mainstream sort of health models'. Indeed, this understanding of the effects of sexual violence in the context of psychological trauma has enabled services and practitioners to challenge 'the pathologising and totalising women and children's experiences as being somehow mental health deficits'. The practitioner who understands trauma understands that even reactions that may appear extreme are 'normal, expected effects of terrible trauma'. The problem's origin shifts from the individual and their perceived internal deficits to an external focus on their experiences of sexual trauma, and it is this that challenges the pathologising practices of medicine and psychiatry.

In the next excerpt, a practitioner explains how this reorientation of the 'problem' affects the way sexual assault practitioners work:

> I mean, so that's also one of the differences between say, for example, the complex trauma and that borderline personality disorder diagnosis is in

> some ways—whether you call it complex sexual assault trauma or borderline personality disorder, there might not be massive differences in how you're going to work with that person towards recovery except that by if you say the person has a borderline personality disorder or some other mental illness, you're saying you're the one that's got the problem, they're saying—whereas if you say you're suffering from complex sexual assault trauma, there's some terrible things going on with you but the reason for that is what's happened to you. And that is a whole different view of the person—it creates a whole stack of different sorts of empathy and it allows you to work with that person in quite a different and more respectful way, and that's really important. (Interview Text No. 1)

Again, the utility of complex trauma lies in the way it enables the shift in the locus of the problem from the personality of the survivor to what has happened to them. Indeed, practitioners constantly identified this capacity for reorienting the problem from the individual to the traumatic experiences as what made complex trauma not only compatible with but an integral part of their feminist framework: 'A feminist perspective specifies that the problem is the sexual assault that has occurred, rather than the problem existing within the survivor as tends to happen with the medical model and diagnosis of BPD' (Interview Text No. 3). This is important, because it enables 'a whole different view of the person' and, by doing so, enables the practitioner to respond with empathy, understanding and respect both for how the client has come to have such difficulties and for their capacity to survive.

Equally significantly, the practitioner draws attention to the fact that the shift from BPD to complex trauma does not necessarily change the types of difficulties with which the person struggles. Regardless of whether their difficulties are framed as BPD or complex trauma, the types of interventions will focus on difficulties such as regulating emotions, tolerating distress, assisting with negotiating relationships and communicating with others. This is important. Medical anthropologist and practising psychotherapist Rebecca Lester (2013), in a nuanced reflection on both the academic and clinical positions on BPD, points out that what can drop from view in feminist critique is the extent to which the diagnostic features of BPD 'are often deeply resonant with clients' daily lived experiences' (p. 71). In making this observation, she is not negating the work of feminist scholars in drawing attention to the problematic ways, at a cultural level, BPD obscures both the social context in which the behaviours arise and the extent to which the diagnostic criteria are based in normative ideas about female behaviour and disposition (p. 71). Nor is she ignoring the disdain, contempt and generally poor treatment meted out by many clinicians who work with this population group. Rather, her concern is that

> feminist critiques have tended to work from the top down; that is, to consider how psychiatric discourses lead clinicians to read women's behavior in certain pejorative ways. What tends to drop out of such analyses is the possibility that many women really do struggle with the behaviors and experiences associated with BPD. (Lester, 2013, p. 73)

The concept of complex trauma as envisioned by Herman and as deployed by practitioners in the NSW sexual assault services sector appears to enable an empathetic acknowledgement of such behaviours and difficulties by understanding them as responses to the abuse to which the client was subjected to through their childhood years. This reorientation, from symptoms of perceived personality deficits to effects of traumatic childhood experiences, enables an appreciation of the extent to which these characteristic difficulties, although now causing considerable problems in the adult survivor's life, nevertheless indicate 'enormous resilience, adaptation, creativity, and a struggle to survive environments that have been invalidating, abusive, or erasing' (Lester, 2013, p. 72).

Moreover, the centring of childhood sexual abuse as the explanatory framework is consistent with the approach adopted in academic feminist critique of BPD (Shaw & Proctor, 2005; Warner, 2009; Warner & Wilkins, 2003). Shaw and Proctor (2005), for example, conceptualise BPD as the last in a long line of historical narratives that aim to dismiss and silence women's attempts to survive and resist oppression and abuse by describing the strategies they use as symptomatic of pathology. Similarly, Warner and Wilkins (2003) argue that 'many of the "symptoms" associated with child sexual abuse (such as deliberate self-harm) are interchangeable with the "symptoms" associated with borderline personality disorder', and go as far as to suggest that 'borderline personality disorder can be understood as the social embodiment of childhood sexual abuse' (pp. 172–173). Drawing on research conducted on the use of the BPD diagnosis in women's secure mental health facilities in the United Kingdom, Warner and Wilkins (2003) argue that one of the many problems with BPD is that it precludes practitioners from considering the underlying cause of the woman's distress. Rather than seeking to understand the impacts of earlier experiences of abuse, the preoccupation remains with identifying and treating symptoms.

This positioning of child sexual abuse as underpinning adult difficulties is not limited to characteristics associated with the BPD diagnosis. The range of symptoms or effects captured in the framework of complex trauma—suicidality, self-harm, relationship problems and alcohol and drug addiction—invites the practitioner to understand a range of different problems through the lens of childhood sexual abuse. This type of positioning occurred repeatedly through the interview texts and is encapsulated in the following excerpt:

> I think, certainly in the last few years where I've done a lot more work with adult survivors—like it's really clear that survivors are vastly overrepresented in all our health care and system, like mental health, drug and alcohol, corrections, child protection and police—like across the board. Survivors are overrepresented and often it's often-untreated traumas that core issue and there's been this very fragmented—all of these issues are impacts and effects of either long-term or short-term trauma and all getting treated as if that's the problem—a drug and alcohol problem, the mental health problem, the homelessness, depression when in actual fact it's untreated trauma that's happening. (Interview Text No. 17)

Indeed, one of the most consistent 'truths' across the interview texts is that the problems 'adult survivors' experience in adulthood are the effects of untreated childhood trauma. The problems with which they present to other services, whether that be drug and alcohol services, mental health services or homelessness services, are symptomatic of the underlying or 'core issue' of untreated childhood trauma. An additional and important issue the practitioner alludes to is the 'fragmented' interventions that often occur when each issue is treated in isolation.

Certainly, when I worked in sexual assault services and within the Australian health service system more generally, I observed some of the less-than-helpful interventions that occur when survivors have to deal with multiple services and workers. The mental health service becomes involved because the woman is struggling with depression, the women's refuge because they are escaping a violent partner, the child protection service because their current circumstances mean there are concerns for the safety and welfare of their children. The concept of complex trauma can provide the type of framework that enables a holistic response that considers the relationship between the person's various difficulties (Davidson, 2007). And for some people, that common link is their struggles with the effects of child sexual abuse. Yet equally, I have worked with survivors of sexual assault who were referred for sexual assault counselling after a suicide attempt, or because of domestic violence, or who were struggling with any number of problems that fit within the gamut of complex trauma but who did not view their current difficulties as caused by or indeed linked to their experiences of childhood sexual victimisation. Rather, this appeared as a framework or interpretation that had been imposed—often by a service provider, or sometimes by a friend or family member. My concern is that this is the type of interpretation that complex trauma invites.

I am not suggesting that people who have experienced sexual victimisation in childhood are not overrepresented in presentations to mental health services or drug and alcohol services, among prison populations or in women's refuges or homeless shelters. Nor am I suggesting that there is no association between childhood sexual abuse and a diverse range of adverse effects in adulthood, including mental and physical health, and social, sexual and interpersonal relationships. This is well established in the research literature; see, for example, Cashmore and Shakel's (2013) evaluation of the Australian and international literature on the long-term effects of childhood sexual abuse. Identifying a trend or an association, however, is different to according it explanatory status, particularly at the level of individual experience. Used prescriptively, this has the capacity to deprive the individual of their own understandings and their own reflective accounts of their life. Used prescriptively, categories and frameworks, whether they be the diagnostic categories of the DSM or the concepts of complex trauma or 'adult survivor', carry the capacity and, in my view, the danger of imposing explanations that may not fit with or reflect the individual's perceptions or understandings of their current problems and distress. Moving beyond the individual lays the potential to produce a problematic category of victim, or survivor, one who is accorded little agency and is able to inhabit a quite circumscribed subject position. The potential for this type of positioning can perhaps be demonstrated via the way complex trauma can be used to frame rape as an effect or consequence of early childhood trauma.

Adults sexually abused in childhood were typically positioned through the interview texts as being significantly more at risk of re-victimisation in adulthood: 'The effects around being able to be ongoing and safe throughout their lives is often an issue—like the re-victimisation rate of people who have been sexually abused is much higher. So quite pervasive effects over a long period' (Interview Text No. 20). Moreover, where the adult survivor had been the victim of a recent assault, the core underlying issue was often understood to be their childhood sexual victimisation. For example, as the practitioner below comments in relation to referrals they received from an adult sexual assault service,

> they offer a couple of sessions to them for their adult rape but then they realise that childhood sexual assault is the core issue so they refer them to us. So we end up seeing people—like lots of people that have been raped but only in the context of childhood sexual assault. (Interview Text No. 8)

The positioning of child sexual assault as the 'core issue' implies that, like drug and alcohol or mental health problems, an experience of adult sexual victimisation functions as a 'symptom' of untreated trauma. The vulnerability of adults sexually abused in childhood to further re-victimisation, understood within this model as a debilitating effect of trauma, appears to be a strategy used by practitioners to ensure the victim was not blamed or held responsible for the abuse. The next excerpt is illustrative of this deployment:

> I think survivors are very vulnerable to re-victimisation and I know people often say, 'Well, she did this' or 'she did that', but it's like a big part often of working with survivors is safety issues. Like really at risk very traumatised people, putting themselves in very, very risky situations where they may be very vulnerable to ongoing abuse. But I see that as an effect of traumatisation as opposed to—as opposed to something that they did that made this person offend. No matter what situation any of us put ourselves in, the offender can always make a choice not to offend. (Interview Text No. 17)

Adult survivors may put themselves in 'very risky situations', but that is an 'effect of traumatisation'. Childhood trauma such as sexual abuse leaves the adult 'at risk', a term used in child protection, of further abuse. The production of the adult survivor as 'vulnerable' appears to function as a mechanism to ensure responsibility is not shifted back onto the victim. The 'cost' to the victim is a passive, almost childlike, positioning. There is little sense of any agency in this representation. The sexual assault may not be about anything the victim did, or how they dressed or behaved, but it does appear, at least in part, about what they lacked. Moreover, the positioning of adult sexual victimisation as a consequence of prior childhood sexual trauma renders less visible the dynamics and concepts of gender, power and structural inequality, and leaves normative and naturalised concepts of sexuality and sexual development unexamined.

Reavey's (2003) empirical research on contemporary professional and everyday discourses of child sexual abuse highlighted the extent to which a causal relationship between past sexual assault and current adult sexual problems, including sexual victimisation, is taken as a given.

Based on interviews with professionals, survivors of child sexual assault and analysis of published literature in the field, including therapeutic, self-help and survivor accounts, the study focused on the production of the woman sexually assaulted in childhood as 'sexual other' in contemporary discourses of child sexual abuse. Her study asked questions about how women's sexuality was understood in relation to experiences of sexual assault in childhood and analysed the types of narratives used to make these representations of women's sexuality appear natural and reasonable (Reavey, 2003).

As Reavey points out, this attribution of difficulties in adult intimate relationships to sexual abuse in childhood is predicated on a particular set of ideas about 'normal' women. It assumes that non-abused women have been allowed to follow a 'normal' developmental pathway to healthy sexuality, an assumption based on a liberal view of sexuality as about individual freedom and choice. Consequently, the problems faced by women sexually assaulted in childhood are understood as 'personal vulnerabilities', the result of the detrimental effects of childhood sexual victimisation. This not only positions the survivor as 'other', as outside the norm, but also obscures gender and the gendered hierarchy of normative heterosexuality and sexual development, such that operation of gendered power in the present lives of 'survivors' is often neglected (Reavey, 2003, pp. 157–160).

Trauma and the Development of the 'Adult Survivor' Self

As a number of feminist post-structural scholars and researchers working in the area of child sexual assault have pointed out, the attribution of problems experienced in adulthood to sexual victimisation in childhood rests on normative assumptions about childhood development associated with developmental psychology (Burman, 2003; Levett, 2003; O'Dell, 2003; Reavey, 2003; Reavey & Brown, 2006, 2007). In this model, where development is understood as a series of linear stages in which childhood is causally related to later life, the abused child does not grow from vulnerable to invulnerable as other children do but remains in a state of vulnerability (O'Dell, 2003). This understanding of child development is evident throughout the interview texts. The trauma experienced during childhood was understood to have 'interrupted development at crucial stages' (Interview Text No. 3), and because of this, key skills required in adult life were not developed. The typical skills lacking related to interpersonal skills and emotional development, 'the interpersonal effectiveness, the distress toleration, the emotion regulation—those sorts of intrapersonal skills and interpersonal skills' (Interview Text No. 3). As this next practitioner explains, trauma experienced in childhood is different because of the way it impacts the 'developing person':

> I think part of it is when it's happened in childhood—trauma that happens in childhood is different because it impacts on the developing person and when its ongoing it has ongoing and accumulative effects. Where if you've got a person who has gotten relatively healthily to adulthood or even late adolescence and then had a traumatic experience or a series of traumatic experiences but they still have something to return to—their memory of what it's like to be reasonably healthy, where somebody who's experienced abuse from an early age, all they have is that—that's life, that's relationships, that's love. (Interview Text No. 5)

However, refracted through the lens of complex trauma, the relationship between adult problems and sexual abuse in childhood rests on a specific psychological theory of child development—attachment theory—coupled with a neurobiological understanding of embodied development. The specific deployment of these concepts became most visible in accounts produced by practitioners of their work with specific clients. The following section lays out how a particular practitioner described working with a client using a trauma model and then uses the trauma theorists identified as influential to illuminate and make sense of the account. This excerpt is typical in that while the intervention focuses on the client's current difficulties, the ideas informing the intervention focus on the client's early childhood.

The practitioner is drawing on her work with a woman who experienced extreme outbursts of anger, the source of which she did not understand but which had previously resulted in episodes of binge drinking where she left the family home for several weeks at a time. The excerpt begins where the practitioner is explaining the effect that understanding her 'triggers' has had on the woman:

> So this amazing breakthrough in her life has been to discover that, the idea of being triggered. She didn't understand that. And the idea of the whole fight or flight thing, the fact that her whole adrenal system's probably really kind of—because she's had a really long, really severe history of trauma, and so the fact that physiologically, her stress levels are probably already—normal is usually down here—she's already probably up here but like she could not understand why she could go—something would happen and she would feel excluded from her partner's family or something would be happening and she would just lose it. And so basically what this kind of—introducing her to the idea of triggers and the fact that having the memory then activates the physiological response, and the emotional response—and the emotional response is—when she was little was too big for her to cope with and now she can't—well if she had, she might end up drinking so that's—it has revolutionised her life. (Interview Text No. 9)

In this scenario, the woman's current problems (the anger, the drinking and the distress) are understood as effects of her sexual victimisation as a child. Her current situation is not the source of her problems but rather 'triggers' her because it is similar in some way to her childhood experiences of abuse—which may, for example, have involved the perpetrator using the common tactic of scapegoating or isolating her from family members. The crucial point in this scenario is that the underlying cause of her reactions—the physiological arousal and emotional responses—is attributed to the trauma of her childhood abuse rather than to her current life, which is understood only as a reminder to trigger rather than the cause of her reactions.

The idea that particular situations 'trigger' the emotional and physiological reactions the victim experienced at the time of the traumatic event is common to both PTSD and 'complex trauma'. The victim is understood to be 'reliving the trauma', which has been recorded as sensory memories and sensations, rather than as verbal narrative (Briere, 2002; Briere & Jordan, 2009; van der Kolk, 1998; van der Kolk et al., 2005). Trauma theorists propose that because adults who experienced childhood sexual abuse were most often abused by someone with whom they had an ongoing close relationship (a parent or close family member), the traumatic re-experiencing is 'triggered' by their adult relationships rather than, as in adult rape, by discreet sensory reminders such as a particular sound or smell (e.g. Briere, 2002; Briere & Spinazzola, 2005; van der Kolk, 1998).

The relational aspect of trauma experienced in childhood is evident through the interview texts. Adult survivors were characterised as having difficulties with trust, in forming social and intimate relationships. Often this was expressed through the idea that adult survivors have trouble with 'attachment'. In this next excerpt, the practitioner highlights the importance of understanding 'trauma and attachment' when working with adults sexually abused in childhood:

> Certainly I developed a much more solid understanding of the importance of trauma and attachment when I started doing more complex work with adult survivors at [name of service], and realising that because abuse—like the idea of abuse as being perpetrated on an otherwise developing child, and usually the person that's abusing them is a key attachment figure—if it's a parent or a family member. (Interview Text No. 15)

In this scenario, the person who abuses the child is described as usually being a 'key attachment figure'. The complexity of the work appears related to the abuse being perpetrated by an attachment figure and the effects of this on the victim's development as a child and, as a consequence, their current adult functioning.

Broadly, attachment refers to a theory of child development that posits that early relationships form the basis of healthy child development. Typically, the focus is the child/parent relationship, with most research concentrating on mothers[8] (Bolen, 2000). The concept of attachment is

[8] The presence of a concept premised on the role and effects of a disrupted or abusive carer relationship is puzzling in a field where the abuse is overwhelmingly perpetrated by men.

key to the internal logic of complex trauma and the types of symptoms associated with it. There are two aspects to this. First, the primary caregiver is essential in modulating the young child's physiological and emotional reactions, which in later years gives them the ability to calm themselves and regulate their emotions. The well-cared-for child experiences small levels of internal discomfort, which over time they learn to tolerate and moderate. The level of distress experienced by young children with abusive caregivers overwhelms their internal resources. The abuse promotes chronic physiological arousal, which the child attempts to modulate by maladaptive means—for example, by inhibiting distress so they lose touch with how they are feeling, by aggression or by dissociation (Briere, 2002; Briere, Hodges, & Godbout, 2010; van der Kolk, 1998). As adults, abused children experience difficulty in regulating emotions and may be seen as moody and emotionally hyper-responsive (Briere, 2002, p. 6).

Second, early attachment relationships are viewed as providing the schema, the internal worldview for how the individual sees themselves and relates to others, and are believed to form the basis of the individual's capacity to form positive adult relationships (Briere, 2002; van der Kolk, 1997). The abused child with an internalised schema based on an abusive relationship is believed to be at increased risk of replicating that relationship in adulthood, either as a victim or as an offender (Bolen, 2000, p. 147). According to Briere (2002), the central mark left by early abuse is negative preverbal assumptions and schema—for example, the belief that the self is bad and others are dangerous. These core schemas affect the individual's ability to form positive relationships as adults, but because they operate at an implicit or non-verbal level, the individual may not be aware of the relationship between their early abuse and current difficulties.

Even if primary carer status is extended to fathers, the theory does not account for the many 'adult survivors' who are not abused by fathers or stepfathers. It may be that the theory of attachment has been extended, or aspects extrapolated in sexual assault knowledge/practices, to include other types of child/adult relationships. As this was not made explicit in the practitioner interview texts, it is not possible to do more than speculate. However, the concept of attachment does appear to contribute further to an individualised understanding of sexual victimisation via the idea that the internalised abusive relationship is replicated in adulthood, and the focus on the maternal caregiver has the potential, whether explicitly or implicitly, to refocus responsibility on mothers.

Moreover, because early traumatic abuse diverts attention away from internal experience and towards the unsafe external environment, the survivor becomes 'other directed' (Briere, 2002, p. 93). Briere (2002) argues that the survivor's external focus makes sense when the environment is dangerous. However, because it interferes with the development of self-awareness, internal security and self-direction, it leaves the individual with impairments in 'self capacities', including difficulty in regulating emotions and with her sense of identity, of what she thinks and feels as opposed to what others think and feel. In Briere's (2002) self-trauma model, traumatic responses are viewed as inborn mechanisms that promote healing rather than as symptoms of pathology. For example, he sees the constant reactivation and then avoidance of traumatic memory as an inherent tendency to 'titrate' or control exposure to traumatic memories and as part of an attempt to heal from traumatic experiences (p. 7).

The self-trauma model (Briere, 2002) works with this tendency to assist the 'survivor' to gradually process and tolerate the memories so they no longer cause overwhelming distress. As part of this process, the model includes the development of 'self capacities' such as learning to regulate emotions and develop a stronger and more positive sense of self. In the self-trauma model, a positive sense of self is facilitated through 'identity training', which uses 'Socratic' questioning to assist the survivor to direct her attention inwards and discover what she thinks and feels. This technique can also be used to address abuse-related 'cognitive distortions' such as the 'survivor' believing they are responsible for the abuse.

Briere's model appears to operate from a stance in which the survivor of childhood abuse is positioned not as exhibiting symptoms of pathology but as demonstrating an inborn capacity to heal from the abuse. The therapist's role is represented as assisting and strengthening this naturally occurring process. Similarly, Herman (1992b, 1997, 2001) understood the symptoms of personality disorders such as BPD not as symptomatic of underlying pathology but as understandable reactions to ongoing experiences of traumatic abuse in childhood. Thus, both theorists can be seen as using the concept of trauma, specifically 'complex trauma', to reposition a disenfranchised victim. The 'adult survivor' who has been misdiagnosed and mistreated as suffering from a pathological condition can, via the concept of 'complex trauma', be positioned as a legitimate victim of abuse who is experiencing legitimate and recognised reactions to that abuse. However, there is also potential in the ideas that make up and underpin 'complex trauma' for the production of, if not pathological then certainly problematic, 'survivor' subject positions. Examples of this were evident in the previous section, where the 'adult survivor' appeared positioned as vulnerable and 'at risk' as a means of countering any belief that she was responsible for her re-victimisation in adulthood.

Conclusion

Through this chapter I have aimed to provide an insight into what the deployment of trauma looks like in the applied context of sexual assault service provision. Through doing so I hope to contribute to shifting the terms of the debate by demonstrating that there are no easy dualisms in which the trauma in work against sexual assault can be positioned as automatically and unproblematically negative—as sure sign of the medicalisation of sexual assault, for example, or as unproblematically positive—as encapsulating a natural, progressive and 'true' account of what sexual violence does to a person. Rather, by focusing on the way trauma is put to work I have attempted to illuminate both its productive and the problematic possibilities. Trauma accomplishes many things for the sexual assault practitioners with whom I conducted my research. It provides a language to convey the violation to the self that lies at the heart of the contemporary experience of sexual violence and to communicate a sense of empathy and understanding of victimising experiences. Mobilising the concept and diagnosis of complex trauma was understood as an enabling device that both guided the practitioners' interventions with adult survivors of childhood sexual abuse and as a strategy with which to advocate against their poor treatment within systems such as mental health services, where survivors are often subject to the prejudicial diagnosis of BPD and where their symptoms are often misunderstood as the cause of the their distress. However, as I laid out, this recourse to childhood trauma as the explanatory tool for problems experienced in adulthood also produces a constrained subject position for the adult survivor, one in which the agency she is afforded can appear troublingly limited. Yet, as Gavey (2003) reminds us, while the uptake of trauma, or aspects of that uptake, in feminist work may appear problematic, this has to be assessed against the alternatives available:

> As actors faced with limitations and opportunities provided by systems not of our own making, political action is inevitably fraught with compromise.

> For one thing, we have to be mindful of what the alternatives are. While the framework of trauma, for instance, might be limiting and problematic in many ways, from a feminist point of view, it has to be seen and judged alongside the other cultural resources that are readily available to children and women for making sense of sexual abuse. That is the victim-blaming, shame-inducing, trivialising, silencing, and threatening discourses through which abuse is perpetuated and ignored. With this in mind, a psychologising ontology of the traumatic effects of sexual abuse might in some cases be extremely liberating. Moreover, feminists such as Judith Butler (1993) have emphasised there is potential for refusal and/or rupture in processes of interpellation. No discourses are totalising, and it is possible that I am overstating the power of psychology and psychological practice. (p. 205)

As Gavey points out, political action always involves compromises. With this in mind, it is important to consider the alternatives for practitioners who work with adults sexually abused in childhood in 'systems not of our own making' and for 'adult survivors' themselves. Moreover, as I go onto discuss in more detail through the next chapter, the discerning way in which practitioners engage with trauma models, concepts and frameworks suggests that there is indeed 'potential for refusal and/or rupture in processes of interpellation' (Gavey, 2003, p. 205).

References

American Psychiatric Association. (2013). *Diagnostic and statistical manual of mental disorders: DSM-5*. Washington, DC: Author.

Bolen, R. (2000). Validity of attachment theory. *Trauma, Violence, Abuse, 1*, 128–153.

Bourke, J. (2009). *Rape: Sex, violence, history*. Berkeley, CA: Counterpoint.

Briere, J. (2002). Treating adult survivors of severe childhood abuse and neglect: Further development of an integrative model. In J. E. B. Myers, L. Berliner, J. Briere, C. T. Hendrix, T. Reid, & C. Jenny (Eds.), *The APSAC handbook on child maltreatment* (2nd ed.). Newbury Park, CA: Sage Publications.

Briere, J., Hodges, M., & Godbout, N. (2010). Traumatic stress, affect dysregulation, and dysfunctional avoidance: A structural equation model. *Journal of Traumatic Stress, 23*(6), 767–774. https://doi.org/10.1002/jts.20578

Briere, J., & Jordan, C. E. (2009). Childhood maltreatment, intervening variables, and adult psychological difficulties in women: An overview. *Trauma, Violence, & Abuse, 10*(4), 375–388. https://doi.org/10.1177/1524838009339757

Briere, J., Kaltman, S., & Green, B. L. (2008). Accumulated childhood trauma and symptom complexity. *Journal of Traumatic Stress, 21*(2), 223–226. https://doi.org/10.1002/jts.20317

Briere, J., & Spinazzola, J. (2005). Phenomenology and psychological assessment of complex posttraumatic states. *Journal of Traumatic Stress, 18*(5), 401–412. https://doi.org/10.1002/jts.20048

Burke, J., Mulder, E., Gravina, J., Walker, H., & Dombrowski, J. (2014). *A best practice manual for specialised sexual, domestic and family violence counselling* (3rd ed.). Drummoyne, NSW: Rape and Domestic Violence Services Australia.

Burman, E. (2003). Childhood, sexual abuse and contemporary political subjectivities. In P. Reavey & S. Warner (Eds.), *New feminist stories of child sexual abuse. Sexual scripts and dangerous dialogues* (pp. 34–51). London: Routledge.

Burstow, B. (2005). A critique of posttraumatic stress disorder and the DSM. *Journal of Humanistic Psychology, 45*(4), 429–445.

Cashmore, J., & Shakel, R. (2013). *The long-term effects of child sexual abuse CFCA paper no 11.* Melbourne: Australian Institute of Family Studies.

Cloitre, M., Courtois, C. A., Charuvastra, A., Carapezza, R., Stolbach, B. C., & Green, B. L. (2011). Treatment of complex PTSD: Results of the ISTSS expert clinician survey on best practices. *Journal of Traumatic Stress, 24*(6), 615–627. https://doi.org/10.1002/jts.20697

Cloitre, M., Garvert, D. W., Brewin, C. R., Bryant, R. A., & Maercker, A. (2013). Evidence for proposed ICD-11 PTSD and complex PTSD: A latent profile analysis. *European Journal of Psychotraumatology, 4*(1), 20706. https://doi.org/10.3402/ejpt.v4i0.20706

Courtois, C., & Ford, J. (2009). *Treating complex traumatic stress disorders: An evidence-based guide.* New York: Guilford Press.

Cvetkovich, A. (2003). *An archive of feelings: Trauma, sexuality, and lesbian public cultures.* Durham, NC: Duke University Pres.

Davidson, J. (2007). *Looking to a future: A research report on the Jacaranda project.* Sydney: Northern Sydney Sexual Assault Service.

ECAV. (2019). *Overview of dialectical behaviour therapy (DBT) in responding to people with complex trauma.* Retrieved from http://www.ecav.health.nsw.gov.au/sexual-assault-courses/

Egan, S. (2016). Sexual assault as trauma: A Foucauldian examination of knowledge practices in the field of sexual assault service provision. *Feminist Review, 112*(112), 95–112. https://doi.org/10.1057/fr.2015.47. [Material reprinted with permission from SAGE Publications].

Fassin, D., & Rechtman, R. (2009). *The empire of trauma: An inquiry into the condition of victimhood* (R. Gomme, Trans.). Princeton, NJ and Oxford: Princeton University Press.

Foucault, M. (1972). *The archaeology of knowledge & the discourse on language* (A. Sheridan, Trans.). New York: Pantheon Books.

Foucault, M. (1988). *Politics, philosophy, culture: Interviews and other writings, 1977–1984* (A. Sheridan, Trans.). New York: Routledge.
Foucault, M. (1998). *The will to knowledge. The history of sexuality: 1* (A. Sheridan, Trans.). London: Penguin Books.
Gavey, N. (2003). Writing the effects of sexual abuse: Interrogating the possibilities and pitfalls of using clinical psychology expertise for a critical justice agenda. In P. Reavey & S. Warner (Eds.), *New feminist stories of child sexual abuse. Sexual scripts and dangerous dialogues* (pp. 187–209). London: Routledge.
Gavey, N., & Schmidt, J. (2011). 'Trauma of rape' discourse: A double- edged template for everyday understandings of the impact of rape? *Violence Against Women, 17*(4), 433–456.
Giourou, E., Skokou, M., Andrew, S. P., Alexopoulou, K., Gourzis, P., & Jelastopulu, E. (2018). Complex posttraumatic stress disorder: The need to consolidate a distinct clinical syndrome or to reevaluate features of psychiatric disorders following interpersonal trauma? *World journal of psychiatry, 8*(1), 12–19. https://doi.org/10.5498/wjp.v8.i1.12
Hall, S. (2004). Foucault and discourse. In C. Seale (Ed.), *Social research methods reader* (pp. 345–349). London: Routledge.
Herman, J. (1992a). Complex PTSD: A syndrome in survivors of prolonged and repeated trauma. *Journal of Traumatic Stress, 5*(3), 377–391. https://doi.org/10.1002/jts.2490050305
Herman, J. (1992b). *Trauma and recovery: The aftermath of violence—From domestic abuse to political terror.* New York: Basic Books.
Herman, J. (1997). *Trauma and recovery: The aftermath of violence—From domestic abuse to political terror.* New York: Basic Books.
Herman, J. (2001). *Trauma and recovery: The aftermath of violence—From domestic abuse to political terror.* London: Pandora.
Herman, J. (2012). CPTSD is a distinct entity: Comment on Resick et al. (2012). *Journal of Traumatic Stress, 25*(3), 256–257. https://doi.org/10.1002/jts.21697
Hunter, S. V. (2010). Evolving narratives about childhood sexual abuse: Challenging the dominance of the victim and survivor paradigm. *The Australian and New Zealand Journal of Family Therapy, 31*, 176–198. https://doi.org/10.1375/anft.31.2.176
Karatzias, T., & Cloitre, M. (2019). Treating adults with complex posttraumatic stress disorder using a modular approach to treatment: Rationale, evidence, and directions for future research. *Journal of Traumatic Stress, 32*(6), 870–876. https://doi.org/10.1002/jts.22457
Karatzias, T., & Levendosky, A. A. (2019). Introduction to the special section on complex posttraumatic stress disorder (CPTSD): The evolution of a disorder. *Journal of Traumatic Stress, 32*(6), 817–821. https://doi.org/10.1002/jts.22476

Kezelman, C., & Stavropolous, P. (2018). *Talking about trauma: Guide to conversations and screening for health and other service providers*. Sydney: Blue Knot Foundation.

Kezelman, C., & Stavropolous, P. (2019). *Practice guidelines for clinical treatment of complex trauma*. Sydney: Blue Knot Foundation.

Kulkarni, J. (2017). Complex PTSD: A better description for borderline personality disorder? *Australasian Psychiatry, 25*(4), 333–335. https://doi.org/10.1177/1039856217700284

Lamb, S. (1999). Constructing the victim: Popular images and lasting labels. In S. Lamb (Ed.), *New versions of victims. Feminists struggle with the concept* (pp. 108–138). New York & London: New York University Press.

Lester, R. J. (2013). Lessons from the borderline: Anthropology, psychiatry, and the risks of being human. *Feminism & Psychology, 23*(1), 70–77. https://doi.org/10.1177/0959353512467969

Levett, A. (2003). Problems of cultural imperialism in the study of child sexual abuse. In P. Leavey & S. Warner (Eds.), *New feminist stories of child sexual abuse. Sexual scripts and dangerous dialogues* (pp. 52–76). London: Routledge.

Mardorossian, C. M. (2002). Towards a new feminist theory of rape. *Signs, 27*(3), 743–775.

Marecek, J. (1999). Trauma talk in feminist clinical practice. In S. Lamb (Ed.), *New versions of victims: Feminist struggle with the concept* (pp. 158–182). New York: New York University Press.

NSW Health. (2020). *Responding to Sexual assault (adult and child) policy and procedures*. Sydney: NSW Health.

O'Dell, L. (2003). The 'harm' story in childhood sexual abuse: Contested understandings, disputed knowledges. In P. Reavey & S. Warner (Eds.), *New feminist stories of child sexual abuse. Sexual scripts and dangerous dialogues* (pp. 131–147). London: Routledge.

Pai, A., Suris, A. M., & North, C. S. (2017). Posttraumatic stress disorder in the DSM-5: Controversy, change, and conceptual considerations. *Behavioral Sciences, 7*(1), 7.

Price-Robertson, R. (2018). *Diagnosis in child mental health: Exploring the benefits, risks and alternatives CFCA paper no. 48*. Melbourne: Australian Institute of Family Studies.

Rape and Domestic Violence Services Australia, (R&DVSA). (2019). *Understanding and responding to complex trauma*. Retrieved from www.rape-dvservices.org.au/training-and-professional-services/for-frontline-workers

Reavey, P. (2003). When past meets present to produce a sexual 'other': Examining professional and everyday narratives of child sexual abuse and sexuality. In P. Reavey & S. Warner (Eds.), *New feminist stories of child sexual abuse: Sexual scripts and dangerous dialogues* (pp. 148–166). London: Routledge.

Reavey, P. (2010). Rethinking agency through materiality. In J. Haaken & P. Reavey (Eds.), *Memory matters. Contexts for understanding sexual abuse recollections* (pp. 131–141). London: Routledge.

Reavey, P., & Brown, S. D. (2006). Transforming past agency and action in the present time: Social remembering and child sexual abuse. *Theory & Psychology, 16*(2), 179–202.

Reavey, P., & Brown, S. D. (2007). Rethinking agency in memory: Space and embodiment in memories of child sexual abuse. *Journal of Social Work Practice, 21*(1), 5–21.

Resick, P. A., Bovin, M. J., Calloway, A. L., Dick, A. M., King, M. W., Mitchell, K. S., … Wolf, E. J. (2012). A critical evaluation of the complex PTSD literature: Implications for DSM-5. *Journal of Traumatic Stress, 25*(3), 241–251. https://doi.org/10.1002/jts.21699

Rose, N. (1996). Critical history and psychology. In C. F. Graumann & K. J. Gergen (Eds.), *Historical dimensions of psychological discourse.* New York: Cambridge University Press.

Roth, S., Newman, E., Pelcovitz, D., van der Kolk, B., & Mandel, F. S. (1997). Complex PTSD in victims exposed to sexual and physical abuse: Results from the DSM-IV field trial for posttraumatic stress disorder. *Journal of Traumatic Stress, 10*(4), 539–555. https://doi.org/10.1002/jts.2490100403

Salter, M., Conroy, E., Dragiewicz, M., Burke, J., Ussher, J., Middleton, W., … Noack-Lundberg, K. (2020). *'A deep wound under my heart': Constructions of complex trauma and implications for women's wellbeing and safety from violence* (Research report, 12/2020). Sydney: ANROWS.

Shaw, C., & Proctor, G. (2005). Women at the margins: A critique of the diagnosis of borderline personality disorder. *Feminism & Psychology, 15*(4), 483–490.

van der Kolk, B. (1997). The psychobiology of posttraumatic stress disorder. *The Journal of Clinical Psychiatry, 58*, 16–24.

van der Kolk, B. (1998). The psychology and psychobiology of developmental trauma. In A. Stoudemire (Ed.), *Human behavior: An introduction for medical students* (Vol. 918, pp. 383–402). Philadelphia, PA: Lippincott, Williams and Wilkins.

van der Kolk, B., Roth, S., Pelcovitz, D., Sunday, S., & Spinazzola, J. (2005). Disorders of extreme stress: The empirical foundation of a complex adaptation to trauma. *Journal of Traumatic Stress, 18*(55), 389–399.

Warner, S. (2003). *Disrupting Identity through Visible Therapy: A Feminist Post-structuralist Approach To Working With Women Who Have Experienced Child Sexual Abuse.* In New Feminist Stories of Child Sexual Abuse. Sexual Scripts and Dangerous Dialogues (pp. 226–247). London: Routledge.

Warner, S. (2009). *Understanding the effects of child sexual abuse: Feminist revolutions in theory, research and practice.* London: Routledge.

Warner, S., & Wilkins, T. (2003). Diagnosing distress and reproducing disorder: Women, child sexual abuse and 'borderline personality disorder'. In P. Reavey & S. Warner (Eds.), *New feminist stories of child sexual abuse: Sexual scripts and dangerous dialogues* (pp. 167–186). London: Routledge.

Wilkin, L., & Hillock, S. (2014). Enhancing MSW students' efficacy in working with trauma, violence, and oppression: An integrated feminist-trauma framework for social work education. *Feminist Teacher, 24*(3), 184–206.

Worrell, M. (2003). Working at being survivors: Identity gender and participation in self-help groups. In P. Leavey & S. Warner (Eds.), *New feminist stories of child sexual abuse. Sexual scripts and dangerous dialogues* (pp. 210–225). London, England: Routledge.

Young, A. (1995). *The harmony of illusions: The invention of post traumatic stress disorder*. Princeton, NJ: Princeton University Press.

CHAPTER 5

Trauma as Feminist Practice

Introduction

In Chapter 4, I demonstrated how sexual assault has been produced as trauma in the field of sexual assault service provision. The focus of this chapter is to both investigate how practitioners have integrated trauma with feminist knowledge practices and understand how trauma, a form of knowledge drawn from medicine and psychiatry, has achieved a position of truth in a feminist field of practice. I begin by tracing the historical trajectory of trauma into feminist work against sexual assault, highlighting that while the uptake in its present iteration—as part of a formalised psychiatric nomenclature—is contentious, the idea that sexual violence causes harm to the victim's psyche has been present in feminism since the second wave.

Moreover, I suggest that the stance taken in most contemporary academic feminist scholarship, that feminist practitioners have passively or unknowingly been co-opted into adopting a trauma model of sexual violence, has rendered invisible the active and knowing way practitioners are capable of negotiating the 'perils' of trauma.

Historicising Trauma

Trauma is a relatively recent psychological concept. Until the late-nineteenth century, the term referred exclusively to physical injuries. The extension of trauma to include psychogenic ailments was enabled through

S. Egan, *Putting Feminism to Work*,
https://doi.org/10.1007/978-3-030-22109-6_5

an analogy that connected the newly discovered effects of surgical shock to effects that could occur due to 'nervous shock' (Young, 1995, p. 66). In the 1860s, John Eric Erichsen, a professor of surgery in London, used the term railway spine to capture his observations of the effects that physical injuries suffered in railway accidents often had on the patient's nervous system (Bourke, 2009, 2012). Erichsen, along with a number of other medical specialists, later revised his ideas on the understanding that fear and psychological shock have the capacity to affect the nervous system independent of any physical injury. Similar discussions took place in the late-nineteenth century in relation to the neuroses suffered by soldiers during military campaigns. Thus, we can trace the lineage of the concept of psychological injury, an injury to the psyche, to the analogy with medical notions of corporal injury, so that we now 'speak as readily of a psychic scar as a physical scare' (Fassin & Rechtman, 2009, p. 284).

Well into the twentieth century, however, trauma remained a 'suspect' condition. As combat neurosis or shellshock, the condition was associated with soldiers in the First and Second World Wars who, it was frequently assumed, were simulating symptoms to avoid returning to the front. The role of any psychiatrist or psychologist involved was to question the credibility of the 'victim' who generally was not considered as such (Fassin & Rechtman, 2009, pp. 4–5). The Vietnam War's aftermath and political mobilisation in support of veterans led to large-scale research studies and treatment centres for veterans. This culminated in the inclusion of psychological trauma as PTSD in DSM-III (1980), the American Psychiatric Association's official nosology (Hunter, 2010; Young, 1995). The major impetus behind DSM-III had been to move away from the psychoanalytic ideas that informed DSM-II towards the implementation of 'objective' diagnostic criteria and the effects of environment on the development of mental illness (Young, 1995). The inclusion of PTSD in DSM-III not only gave the condition diagnostic legitimacy but also removed any lingering vestiges of thinking that viewed trauma reactions as the result of pre-existing personality or character weakness. Rather, in DSM-III, the aetiology of trauma is externally located, the consequence of distressing events that lay outside the usual range of human experience. Although there have been some modifications with each version of the diagnostic manual, this distinctive feature, where the aetiology of PTSD is understood as caused by external events, remains consistent (American Psychiatric Association, 2000, 2013; Pai, Suris, & North, 2017).

The study of psychological trauma is now a well-established field of research and practice, with a proliferation of specialised journals, research centres, societies, websites, support centres, experts and popular books on trauma (Fassin & Rechtman, 2009). These include The Trauma Center in the United States (www.traumacenter.org), the *Journal of Traumatic Stress* (www.onlinelibrary.wiley.com/journal/15736598), the International Society for Traumatic Stress Studies (www.istss.org), the Australasian Society for Traumatic Stress Studies (www.astss.org.au) and the Centre for Interdisciplinary Trauma Research in New Zealand (niphmhr.aut.ac.nz/research-centres/interdisciplinary-trauma-research-centre).

Sexual Violence and Trauma

As Bourke (2012) demonstrates, the harm of sexual violence has not always been understood as psychological injury or trauma. For working class women in nineteenth-century United Kingdom and United States, the harm of sexual violence was to her social standing, her class or respectability, and earning capacity. The forensic texts of the time located the harm in the topography of the body; the victim experienced convulsions, hysteria or epilepsy because of the loss of her 'fair name and chastity'. Women's accounts placed emphasis on physical injury or on the threat of pregnancy, and focused much more on the pain of defloration and ejaculation than do contemporary accounts. Thus, rape was understood—in those instances where it was acknowledged as such—as an attack on the victim's social identity rather than as an attack on the individual's sexual identity or inner self (Bourke, 2012, p. 40). In the mid-twentieth century, the little that was written in medical and criminal science texts continued to focus on physical injury, pregnancy and the risk of sexually transmitted disease (Bourke, 2012, p. 30).

Indeed, Bourke (2012) points out that the narrative of psychological trauma did not enter professional understandings of rape until over a century after the discovery of 'nervous shock'. Bourke (2012), in her analysis of the substantial lag in conceptualising rape as a traumatic event, not surprisingly highlights the public nature of the types of events designated as traumatic. Events such as military conflict and railway accidents associated with industrialisation were 'unnatural' events, the occurrence of which was outside the victim's control.[1] Rape, however, was the outcome of a 'natural' but thwarted biological sex drive, a 'private' misfortune in which the victim was typically seen as complicit. Consequently, as discussed in Chapter 3 the little research that did focus on sexual violence apportioned blame to the victim—for example, Amir's (1968) concept of 'victim precipitated rape'. It was not until the 1970s that some medical and psychological literature began to draw attention to the victim's experience. For example, by 1974, psychiatric nurse Ann Burgess and sociologist Lynda Holmstrom (1974) had published their groundbreaking US study on the detrimental psychological and emotional consequences of rape. The research described the pattern of acute behaviour and emotional and psychological effects they had identified in rape victims seen through the emergency department of a Boston hospital and which they referred to as 'rape trauma syndrome'.

Entry of Trauma into Feminist Approaches to Sexual Violence

The trajectory of psychological trauma into feminist work against sexual violence appears to have origins in the second-wave feminist movement (e.g. Haaken, 1999; Levett, 2003; Mardorossian, 2002). Mardorossian (2002) contends that, in the US context, second-wave feminists initiated the focus on the psychological effects of power, which she argues has remained the accepted approach to the study of the effects of sexual

[1] In the field of nineteenth-century psychoanalysis, some did accord sexual abuse in childhood a role in the development of later trauma reactions; however, as Bourke (2012) points out, these ideas could not be 'easily mapped onto women who had been raped in adulthood' (p. 36). Freud's 'seduction hypothesis', for example, rested on the supposition that trauma reactions or hysteria were caused by memories of abuse that were usually triggered in adulthood by some type of non-traumatic incident (Bourke, 2012, p. 36). However, experience of sexual abuse at the time it occurred was not considered to cause traumatic reactions, as the child victim was believed incapable of grasping its significance. Consequently, this theory did little to account for the reactions of adult women who, as 'sentient beings', were well able to grasp the significance of their experience of rape (Bourke, 2012). Moreover, as is well known, Freud's seduction hypothesis was short lived as he replaced it with the idea that women's accounts of childhood sexual abuse were nothing more than fantasies. In addition, some psychoanalysts such as the French neurologist Jean-Martin Charcot believed traumatic reactions (then referred to as hysteria or nervous disorders) to be hereditary in origin. Although aware that his patients had often experienced earlier rape or child sexual abuse, these experiences were considered at most a 'trigger' for a pre-existing weakness.

violence. She identifies 'consciousness raising' as an early articulation of the feminist focus on the interior psyche and the effects of sexual violence on the psyche.[2] Levett (2003), discussing the effect trauma knowledge/practices have had on sexual assault work (in Anglophone countries), says feminists initially used the concept metaphorically to communicate that, like the body, the mind or 'mental sense of self' could be injured.[3] However, she argues that in contemporary use, trauma has come to denote damaging effects that are presented factually, as in 'broken bones', and are routinely elicited as 'clinical evidence' (Levett, 2003, p. 56).

Haaken and Lamb (2000, p. 1010) suggest the late 1980s as the point by which, in the United States, this general focus on the internal psyche had shifted to the more specific concept of trauma as a discrete set of psychological symptoms and effects. They suggest restrictions on mental health insurance coverage played a part in this shift in the United States, so that feminist practitioners used lists of psychological trauma symptoms to argue for access to therapy and to better insurance benefits for victims of sexual and domestic violence. Within the US women's movement, the work of Judith Herman, a feminist psychiatrist, appears to have been particularly influential (Fassin & Rechtman, 2009, pp. 78–78). In her foundational text *Trauma and Recovery: The Aftermath of Violence, From Domestic Abuse to Political Terror,* Herman (1992) proposed private harms such as sexual and domestic violence should be understood as traumatic events in the same way public forms of violence such as war and political terrorism have come to be understood. This positioning gave feminists a means to counterclaims that the reactions of women to sexual violence were somehow indicative of a pre-existing neurosis or individual fragility. Rather, as PTSD, their reactions could be understood as normal and expected reactions to what had been done to them (Fassin & Rechtman, 2009). Herman explicitly situated herself and her work as part of the second-wave feminist movement, arguing that achieving social and political recognition for victims of 'trauma'—whether as victims of war or of

[2] Similarly Thomson (2006 cited in Crook, 2018) points out that while the British women's movement positioned itself in opposition to and as an alternative to psychiatry it was never the less able to appropriate and use the concept of the emotional and psychological self, via the concept of consciousness and the practice of consciousness raising.

[3] Florence Rush (1980), for example, used the x-ray evidence that had formed part of the 'discovery' of battered baby syndrome in the 1960s as an analogy to explain the harm of the psychological trauma experienced by child victims of sexual assault.

gender violence—could only happen in the context of a strong political movement.

Commenting on the New Zealand context, Gavey (2003) identifies the 1990s as the period during which the 'trauma model' became formalised into its contemporary form 'as a framework for conceptualising the psychological impact of sexual abuse' (p. 200), although she makes the point that prior to this, it had existed as an informal or implied framework in sexual assault work. Nancy Whittier (2009), in a comprehensive empirical study of the politicisation of child sexual assault in the United States from the 1970s onwards, identifies the 1990s as the period in which the feminist movement embraced the 'science' of traumatic memory as a strategy to counter the claims of proponents of false memory syndrome (FMS). The idea that delayed recall of early traumatic experiences is a consequence of the way traumatic memory is encoded in sensory (e.g. visual, aural or bodily) sensations provided a powerful tool to counter accusations beginning in the early 1990s from proponents of FMS that women were fabricating memories of child sexual assault (Whittier, 2009). Regardless of any national variations in the historical trajectory of trauma, there appears a consensus that trauma has assumed a hegemonic position in feminist work against sexual violence assault (Hunter, 2010; Lamb, 1999; Mardorossian, 2002; Marecek, 1999).

Much of the concern and critique, as I discussed in the previous chapter, has focused on trauma in its present iteration—as part of a formalised psychiatric nomenclature and a diagnostic tool. The trauma model is viewed as evidence of the medicalisation of feminist practice, with the conceptual framework operating using the same logic as psychopathology: specifically, that it works based on a simple 'cause and effect' explanation and through doing so reduces women's experiences into a uniform set of symptoms (Marecek, 1999, p. 165). Indeed, many of the concerns about depoliticisation (Bumiller, 2008; Burstow, 2003, 2005), individualisation (Lamb, 1999; Mardorossian, 2002; Marecek, 1999) and therapeutisation (Cvetkovich, 2003; Stark, 2007) can be traced to concern about the place and influence of trauma discourse.

Yet, there seems a subtle dichotomisation in the positioning of the concept of trauma and its deployment by second-wave feminists as metaphor and the positioning of trauma as a 'clinical' concept in the knowledge/practices of contemporary feminist practitioners (Levett, 2003, pp. 55–56). Whether understood as a metaphor to denote injury to the psyche or a set of diagnosable symptoms, the concept of psychological trauma is premised on an understanding of the person as an individualised and internalised self (Rose, 1996).

This type of representation appears present in the position taken by some feminists in which, despite the critique of PTSD, the more metaphorical relationship between trauma and sexual assault is represented as a somewhat naturalised given. Terms such as 'incest trauma' (Hart, 1998, p. 200), 'personal trauma history' (Burstow, 2015, p. 239) and 'trauma survivor' (Wilkin & Hillock, 2014, p. 200) occur throughout this work. Feminist practitioners are referred to as 'trauma practitioners' (Burstow, 2003, p. 1300), victims of rape as 'survivors of trauma' (Hart, 1998, p. 182) and the terms violence and trauma appear interchangeably in some work, for example, Wilkin and Hillock (2014, p. 200).

In this genre of critique, perhaps best encapsulated by the work of radical feminist and anti-psychiatry critic Bonnie Burstow (2015), the concept of psychological trauma is not dismissed; rather, the formalisation as a diagnosis and set of symptoms subject to psychiatric intervention is the focus of critique. Arguing that conceptualising the psychological effects of sexual violence as symptoms produces them as deficits to be fixed, Burstow (2003, 2005) proposes that these effects instead be understood as strategies the victim has used to survive. Understood as survival strategies rather than symptoms of a psychiatric disorder enables the enormous strength and resilience of victims and survivors to be acknowledged both by themselves and by others. I am not suggesting that promoting the resilience of survivors of sexual violence is not a positive move, or that reframing the diagnostic criteria of PTSD as survival strategies does not play an important role. For example, as discussed in the previous chapter, the practitioners identified the shift from borderline personality to complex trauma as significant for similar reasons. The types of difficulties (whether designated as symptoms, effects or survival strategies) the individual struggles with remain similar, but the understanding of the person shifts so that they are no longer viewed as the source of their problems. What is important to though and does not appear acknowledged by Burstow (2003, 2005) is that the concept of trauma she promotes, relies on and is underpinned, in fact, by the psychologising ontology of which she is most critical.

Analysis of how trauma has achieved hegemony in the field of sexual violence often centres on the perceived weakness of the contemporary feminist movement (Lamb, 1999; Levett, 2003; Mardorossian, 2002; Marecek, 1999; O'Dell, 2003). Indeed, Mardorossian (2002) goes so far as to assert that 'trauma talk' has not only reduced victims to a state of 'agentless interiority' but has contributed to 'refashioning the feminist movement itself' (p. 768). She argues that victims, who in earlier years were actively involved in political activism, have been relegated to the backdrop of the feminist movement. Political activism, when it does occur, she suggests, has predominantly become the domain of professionals such as sexual assault counsellors who organise, advocate and speak on behalf of sexual assault victims whose vulnerability and harm precludes their own activism.

This professionalisation of organisations working against sexual assault is often understood as having played a key role in the uptake of trauma and the concordant diminution of grassroots activism. By professionalisation, I mean the transition from grassroots collectives often organised by feminist activists on a volunteer basis to a service-provider model that employs professionally qualified staff and is either provided or funded by government resources. For example, Marecek (1999), in her analysis of trauma's popularity with the feminist therapists interviewed for her research, suggests that the therapists may have 'consciously or unconsciously' modelled their practices on high-status professions like medicine and bio-medicine. Similarly, Mardorossian (2002) suggests, 'We have reverted to a 19th charity model whereby privileged women are seen as better able to help victims cope with and make sense of their experiences' (p. 768). Victims who once actively participated in the running of services are now seen as so irremeably shaped by their traumatic experiences that they are able to do little other than cope with their inner turmoil.

One of the aspects I find troubling about such feminist critique is the way practitioners are positioned as having been co-opted into or as having passively absorbed medical and scientific 'expertise' in ways that place them outside the politics, values and practices of feminism. Moreover, practitioners' views, reflections and experiences are often absent from such accounts. Through this chapter, I explore and aim to bring practitioners' perspectives to the forefront. Trauma made 'sense' to the practitioners with whom I conducted my research and was represented consistently as both compatible with their feminist practices and as part of their established practices of enabling clients to regain power and control. As laid out in the previous chapter, trauma was understood as a form of knowledge that, by normalising adult survivors' reactions, had enabled practitioners and services to advocate against the pathologisation and poor treatment of victims within the mental health system. Without negating the problematic aspects of this deployment, I want to explore now how practitioners make sense of the place of trauma in their work. What has it enabled them to do? Has it changed their work? Do they have any reservations?

Exploring the Compatibility of Feminism and Trauma

In this section, I draw on reflective accounts contained in the interview texts as well as examples of interventions with specific clients that practitioners used to explain and elaborate their points. Practitioners who worked at the most localised level of the field of sexual assault service provision appeared to have utilised trauma knowledge to fill a gap in feminist knowledge/practices. While not the only deployment, trauma seemed to have provided a set of 'technical' skills and 'practical' knowledge that enabled practitioners who intervened at the most immediate level to respond directly to problems that victims of sexual assault brought to counselling, such as the distress caused by constant nightmares or flashbacks of the abuse.

It was the neurobiological aspects of trauma that appeared most frequently deployed as enabling strategies, which were used to assist the victim to understand and thus regain power and control. This knowledge was used most explicitly to assist victims and survivors with myriad material bodily problems that they presented to services. For example, victims may have been dealing with nightmares, insomnia, hyper-alertness, intrusive memories and debilitating effects on daily living.

Practitioners were quite aware of the seeming incongruence of drawing on the work of predominantly male trauma experts, psychiatrists and neuroscientists, as this practitioner points out, reflecting on the changes she had observed over an extensive career working in Australian sexual assault services:

> And here we find ourselves primarily consulting John Briere and Colin Ross and Judith Herman—where in our early days we wouldn't have dared talked to a male psychiatrist about how to effectively work with women survivors of sexual abuse. It was very polarised and I think a very mainstream medical model and a feminist model would have been very critical of each other. (Interview Text No. 19)

These women had been well 'schooled' in feminism. Many had initially encountered feminist ideas and theories through their university studies; some had taken women or gender studies subjects as electives, while others spoke of the influence of feminist academics who had taught in their 'home' departments. Others, typically those with long work histories in the sector, reflected on the ways they had learnt about feminism 'on the job' through the daily processes involved in working in feminist organisations. The synchronicity between their initial interest in feminism and their work against sexual violence was palpable during the interviews. In the words of this interviewee, it was 'a natural kind of organic thing that went with each other. The choice of work and the interest [in feminism] naturally went together' (Interview text No. 15).

Working in a sexual assault service was a place where it was 'very easy to be a feminist' (Interview Text No. 4). Moreover, there was a sense of pride about the place that second-wave feminism and feminists had played in the development of a sexual assault services sector in Australia. They were, as one participant put it, 'a child of the feminist movement'.

Yet through the interviews, there was at times dissatisfaction levelled at some aspects of feminism and feminist approaches to sexual and gendered violence: at the limitations of a highly politicised feminism dedicated to achieving change in the broad-based structural inequalities that enable sexual violence to continue. It was not, as I hope I have amply demonstrated through the previous chapter, that such analysis had been rejected, nor that the pressing need for significant social change was not keenly felt. Rather, it was that such analysis, in and of itself, had proved inadequate to the task of assisting them with the very concrete and embodied problems with which victims and survivors presented to services on a daily basis.

In this next somewhat wry account, the practitioner encapsulates, with a degree of good humour, some of the limitations she encountered in utilising principles of feminist theories, practices and principles in her counselling work.

> I think for me a big shift very early on was the idea that you just let—you want to validate the woman and the client's position as expert on their own story and on their own lives to the point where sometimes we're just sitting there doing a bit of reflective listening. And not wanting to pathologise the experience, and putting it in—locating it in a political and social context, not wanting to take over and acknowledging—a huge amount of acknowledging—of the power relationship of therapy and the counsellor being in

> the power position. And doing all of this while this person's got symptoms of PTSD. And I think this has been a big shift—that people come to therapy with really significant problems and not just because they might decide to tell someone that they were sexually abused but [because of] the impacts and effects and the traumatisation. (Interview Text No. 17)

As she goes on to explain, it is not that she is no longer mindful of the importance of the person's understanding of their needs and of their own life. Nor is she dismissing the importance of acknowledging the power imbalance in the client–counsellor relationship or of the centrality of understanding sexual violence as a social and political problem. Indeed, this worker had been highly involved in political and social change activism for many years. What she is suggesting, however, is that this had not proved sufficient in assisting her to work with survivors to help alleviate the emotional, psychological and bodily reactions to trauma. A broad-based political analysis, however sophisticated and nuanced, does not necessarily help at the coalface in those situations where you are the telephone crisis counsellor and the woman (or man) on the other end of the phone is dissociating or experiencing flashbacks to the abuse or is exhausted from nightmares (Interview Text No. 12).

Yet there was an element of caution or wariness evident in some interviews about potentially negative outcomes of neurobiological understanding of the traumatic effects of sexual violence. In the next excerpt, the practitioner reflects on the longstanding concern by feminists of not pathologising sexual violence and the role the medical model has played in that process.

Practitioner:	I was thinking also we used to be very afraid of pathologising sexual assault.
Interviewer:	In what sort of ways?
Practitioner:	Well, I suppose, the medical model of victims is that sexual assault leaves them incapacitated, I suppose. I think, with this neurobiology stuff, it's sort of—it does recognise that there is some real harm that has happened to someone, to their bodies, to their beings. But, it's important not to buy too much into that as well, because people also have agency and they always have capacity to recuperate and to do things that like helping them as well.

Interviewer: So how do you manage that within your feminist framework? How do you manage that balance?

Practitioner: Well I see—I just see that some people are traumatised and some people aren't. And if a person is traumatised then it's not necessarily—it's something that is about harm, bodily harm and it is something that has to be healed in a way and that's very possible but it still doesn't leave the person without any control. And being acted on. (Interview Text No. 27)

The practitioner identifies what she sees as the positive aspects of the 'neurobiology stuff'. She points to the importance the role of neurobiology has in facilitating recognition of the embodied effects of traumatic reactions to sexual violence. It does harm 'to their bodies [and] to their beings'. This bodily harm refers to the way in which trauma registers in the body as well as in the psyche of the individual: in the heightened startle response and the physiological arousal experienced in response to sensory based memories and reminders of the abuse. This is significant because it points to a shift from understanding trauma as a psychological concept (in the mind) to one that through a neurological framework is able to articulate a relationship between body and mind (being). Yet there is a recognition that with its origins in the 'medical model', this could lead to sexual assault victims being pathologised or treated as 'incapacitated'. Rather, she suggests that while neurobiology has a place in sexual assault work, it is important 'not to buy too much into that' because sexual assault does not leave people 'being acted on'; they still have agency and still have control.

The next sequence of excerpts are illustrative of the ways practitioners have actively integrated feminist and trauma knowledge/s in a way that makes trauma compatible with feminist discourses of sexual violence. In the following case scenario, the practitioner lays out how she uses her understanding of the brain, traumatic memory and PTSD to enable a client to gain a sense of psychological and emotional safety by gaining some control over her traumatic reactions. In this scenario, the woman had been subject to abuse by her partner for many years, and her daily life and functioning had come to be plagued by distressing flashbacks and nightmares to this abuse. This excerpt, presented in two parts, begins with the practitioner explaining her understanding of the concept of traumatic memory and its bodily effects.

> The parts of the brain that are most affected following a traumatic event are the imagery parts of the brain that are actually highlighted in—the chemical produced through PTSD shuts down the cognitive functions and the verbal functions but provides more stimulation and a greater amount to the imagery side, which is why flashbacks and nightmares are such a powerful part of post-traumatic stress disorder. And so it's about harnessing what is already developing, extra senses and so harnessing that part of the brain, the imagery part of the brain—the brain fundamentally doesn't know the difference between what it imagines and what is. The brain will still—so a flashback can be experienced as—that it's actually happening—the body has the same reaction. (Interview Text No. 29)

As discussed in Chapter 4, traumatic memory is understood as stored in the right sphere of the brain and recalled as images and sensations; because of this, it is experienced by the victim as if the traumatic event is happening again (van der Kolk, 1994, 1997, 2000, 2004, 2015; van der Kolk et al., 1996). While explicit (cognitive) memory encoded in the hippocampus which turns raw sensory data into a coherent narrative, traumatic memories often remain in the limbic system in this raw sensory form. Reminders of the abuse trigger these memories along with the emotional responses and body reactions (the increase in adrenaline and cortisol and subsequent increased heartrate and blood pressure) that make it feel to the person as if the trauma is happening all over again[4] (van der Kolk, 2015).

This knowledge of the person feeling and experiencing the same sensations and 'bodily reaction' in a way that feels as if it 'is actually happening' again now helps give a context to and an understanding of the level and nature of the distress. It is experienced not merely as a narrative memory, if distressing, located in time past, but also as a visceral sensation as if it is happening right now, in the present. The practitioner goes on to explain how she uses this 'knowledge' as a strategy to enable her clients to gain a sense of their own power; she explains how she 'harnesses' or uses this knowledge of traumatic memory in her counselling work.

[4] The introduction of functional Magnetic Resonance Imaging (fMRI), technology has increasingly enabled researchers to examine the effects of trauma on the brain. For example, fMRI scans have shown how sensory reminders of the traumatic event result in elevated activity in these parts of the brains (van der Kolk, 2015). Some of the changes in the brain caused by traumatic experiences such as increased activity in the amygdala, seem to occur regardless of whether the individual has symptoms of PTSD or not (see for example a meta-analysis of fMRI studies conducted by Stark et al. (2015).

> So the idea is that we can imagine a different outcome—that we can see ourselves as being powerful. That we can see ourselves as being safe. And so that when a negative image begins to start, people are learning to control the images and are able to change them.… They're able to touch what safety looks like in a safe controlled environment with someone guiding them. So when they go back and they're doing their ordinary life, when things begin to feel unsafe they can work with the images of being safe. It's a very simple kind of—these are the parts of the brain that are so active following assault, so it's about tuning in, using the assets that are there and that are often experienced as a negative. (Interview Text No. 29)

For example, the practitioner explained how the woman discussed above had learnt to replace the 'negative images' of her abuse with an image of a real experience where she had felt safe and secure. This is important as it means that not only an image or cognitive memory is evoked, but also the feelings, emotions and sensations that go with that memory. This is a way of working with trauma that goes beyond psychological effects and begins to work with the embodied effects of abuse and trauma. Experienced first in the safety and context of a therapeutic setting, the survivor is then able to use this strategy in their 'ordinary life', 'when things begin to feel unsafe'. This kind of practice can be understood as an enabling practice, one that assists sexual assault victims to gain some control over reactions that are experienced as real and often quite frightening. In this way, the deployment of this type of trauma knowledge acts as an enabler of the feminist counselling principle of working with victims and survivors to regain the power and control lost through the experience of sexual victimisation.

This can be an important part of communicating a sense of empathy with the person, to begin to build a trusting relationship. In the next part, the practitioner goes on to explain what she sees as the importance of this feminist–trauma framework.

> To have someone who does understand that is like gold because that allows them to be able to express it without feeling like they've failed, that they're stupid. That's what they often say—it's like magic. 'Oh you know what I'm talking about'. I think people, if they understand that something has happened to them and it is trauma—which is an emotional psychological thing and it's about really being incredibly afraid and fearing and to understand what happens in that, actually helps the person to understand what's going

on and become more able to take charge again of themselves. Or at least feel like they get a picture, give some control, I suppose. A sense of understanding. Yeah. (Interview Text No. 27)

Working with someone who understands what they are 'talking about' is an important part of building a sense of trust and in communicating empathy. Understanding trauma can play an integral role in enabling a victim to start to regain a sense of the power and control—over their minds, their emotional responses and in regaining a sense of bodily integrity—that victims often report have been diminished through their experiences of sexual violence (Brison, 1999, 2002). The trauma framework is important because it means the victim feels understood and because they know they are with someone who understands, are able to express their feelings and reactions without feeling 'like they've failed, that they're stupid'. Understanding trauma, and understanding their reactions as trauma reactions, enables victims of sexual assault to 'take charge' of themselves again and gives back 'some control' (Interview Text No. 27).

Enabling Control Through a Framework of Safety

The importance and emphasis on the survivor's safety and the counsellor's role in that process is apparent through the interview texts and is a characteristic feature of trauma-focused models and interventions. Herman's (2001, 2015) three-stage therapeutic model focuses on safety, remembering, and mourning and reconnection. The foundational work is in establishing the survivor's physical and psychological safety, ensuring they are physically safe from further abuse and by assisting them to establish control over their emotional and psychological reactions so that they do not become completely overwhelmed or re-traumatised when recounting their abuse. Similarly, in Briere's (2002; Briere & Scott, 2006) self-trauma model, the counsellor works with the survivor to develop and strengthen capacities such as learning to regulate emotions and attain a more positive sense of themselves so that they are gradually able to cope with their memories of abuse in a way that promotes healing rather than further harm.

The aim is that over time the abusive experiences become integrated as a facet of the person's life, that they are able to say, 'Yes that happened to me, but it's part of my life. It's not what I am or who I am' (Interview Text No. 11). Rather than a cathartic 'get it all out' approach, the counsellor may slow the person down, perhaps suggest they do not try to tell too much in one session. It is about processing and integrating the traumatic experiences, not about 'reliving the trauma' (Interview Text No. 11). The counsellor has a 'responsibility to always ensure that the process is safe' and be mindful of not wanting to 'do anything that would be ineffective or contribute to [making someone] unsafe' (Interview Text No. 10). On this basis, they have a responsibility to share with the client what they know about trauma and its effects, to be able to explain, 'This is what I know and this is why I'm doing this' (Interview Text No. 14). It means your 'expertise as a counsellor sits alongside your client's knowledge and expertise' (Interview Text No. 14).

The following excerpt is illustrative of the compatibility practitioners see between feminism and trauma models and how they integrate feminism and trauma knowledge. The first part begins with a discussion of Briere's (Briere & Scott, 2006, 2014) trauma model.

> So sometimes, when Briere might talk about, he will really strongly talk about going with the client at their pace and their time in a sense and that they will be the expert on, as long as you are taking responsibility as the therapist to be putting in a safe framework around all of this. That's very similar to the feminist model so they're not really at loggerheads. He's got more of a scientific—he kind of I suppose will go into the neurobiological aspects of why someone might be having flashbacks and how traumas—why talking about something actually helps traumatic memory—does it help it and to help it, what would you need to do? So he kind of gets into a little bit more of the technical, which isn't at odds with feminism, it's just feminism doesn't necessarily go the neurobiological route. (Interview Text No. 23)

In this account, the practitioner has identified a compatibility between Briere's emphasis on the counsellor 'going with the client at their pace' and a feminist way of working. Briere's work appears to provide some 'technical' detail and explanation about traumatic memory and the neurobiology of people's reactions. However, she is clear that this does not put it 'at odds with feminism'. In the next part, the practitioner provides an example of how she integrates trauma and feminism in her practice.

> So, yeah, I find it's that thing of being able to just pull out when you're with someone, being able to pull out from the bag of tricks what's fitting. So if that person is really struggling with 'I don't understand why I'm sitting at work, nothing's reminding me of this and then I get this flashback', then

> you pull in more on Briere's stuff. If I'm working with the woman I was describing before, who had a lifetime of sexual assault, she's losing her job from a very high-powered role as a woman. She wanted to talk about the attack, and felt like 'was he trying to bring me down because I was more senior to him'. So then, I'm really drawing on the feminist ideas more strongly, plus some trauma. So it's that thing of being able to pull out whatever [you need] at the time. (Interview Text No. 23)

Again, the practice centres on what the client is struggling with and with the issues about which she wishes to talk. In one scenario, the issue required trauma knowledge, and in the other, feminist knowledge. The practitioner's 'bag of tricks' needs to be varied enough that she has available the knowledge and skills that 'fit' with the individual needs of clients.

Trauma and Crisis Work

Understanding the effects of trauma is particularly important in the crisis work undertaken by sexual assault services. In some services, such as R&DVSA, this means workers are rostered on shifts in order to provide 24-hour crisis telephone counselling. In the NSW Health sexual assault services, the crisis role extends to and often focuses on coordinating the medical response to victims, many of whom contact the service in the initial aftermath of the assault, and often are brought in by the police to whom they have reported the assault.[5] In situations where the victim decides to go ahead with a medical examination, the counsellor's role includes eliciting at least a rudimentary account of what has happened (when, where, who, what) before the medical examination. Often referred to as the medicolegal context of sexual assault work, these notes, along with the medical examiner's notes, form part of the forensic medical examination protocol and are included as part of the kit released to the police. In cases that proceed to court, the forensic kit, including the medical and counselling notes, form part of the evidence presented to the court.

[5] The only service that does not provide a 24-hour crisis response is the community-based CASACS. Rather, in the NGO sector, R&DVSA has the responsibility of running a 24-hour crisis telephone line. NSW Health sexual assault services provide a 24-hour crisis response, which in addition to crisis counselling includes a medical service. As I have discussed in Chapter 3, these latter services provide forensic medical examinations to both child and adult victims.

In such situations, it is crucial that the counsellor has a solid grasp of the fragmented way traumatic experiences are often recalled, as this practitioner, the manager of a major metropolitan Sydney service, explains:[6]

> We know then how to help someone. What to do and what not to do. Not to be expecting—like I said earlier, not to expect someone to be able to just give us this great narrative of what happened to them because we understand that a major shock to someone's system will mean that they are not going to be able to recall all of this really freely. It might be fragmented, it might—they might remember sensory sort of stuff more than a narrative or they might only remember visual things but have no feeling. You know that kind of very fragmented sense of what happened and to me is very normal way of remember trauma. If you understand that, I think it helps you to understand the ways that people present. (Interview Text No. 23)

This is important. It is important because the counsellor needs to understand to understand that the profound effects the traumatic experience, 'the shock to someone's system' (Interview Text No. 23) has on how they recall about the experience, on their emotional reactions (or lack of) to the abuse and to their capacity to communicate this. As the practitioner points out, they know not to expect a chronological linear narrative and that a fragmentary sensory recall is 'a 'very normal way to remember trauma' (Interview Text No. 23).

The substantial neuroscientific research in this area suggests this type of fragmentary recall, sometimes referred to as 'flashbulb moments' is a typical outcome of the body's stress response. Often details that occurs at the beginning the traumatic event can be remembered quite vividly while later details are fuzzy, indistinct or missing (Diamond, Campbell, Park, Halonen, & Zolad, 2007; Schwabe, 2017). Some research suggests the adrenaline release that occurs in response to stress initially enables recall but as it continues to flood the system comes to impairs memory encoding in the hippocampus (Haskell & Randall, 2019). Details that are remembered will be those that were central to the victim's experience while the peripheral detail may not be remembered or may be inconstant. This is important because the details that were central to their experience may not be details such as what the assailant was wearing, the layout of a room in which the abuse occurred. Rather the person may vividly recall the detail

[6] In most services, managers continue to be involved in direct client work including taking part in the crisis roster.

of a bedspread or cushion if that was what they focused on in order to try to cope with the experience. The person may not be able to provide a clear narrative or have a time sequence chronological recall bur may be able to describe at least parts of the experience experientially, particular sounds or smells or images. In addition, a victim who has a freeze response[7] may dissociate during the assault meaning that they may not feel their bodily responses during the assault may not remember parts of the experience. People who have this response often report feeling detached from their emotions, as if they are in a trance or that the situation feels unreal. They may experience periods where they are unable to move or where they feel faint and their body limp (Kozlowska, Walker, McLean, & Carrive, 2015). While the freeze response inhibits movement, the release of neurohormones such as adrenaline and cortisone brings about a state of hyper focus such that minute of details (design of a bed cover) may be recalled but the larger context (room layout) may not have been noticed.

Having access to this type of knowledge and understanding the nature of traumatic memory is especially important in the often pressure-driven environment of crisis work. It is vital that victims are given the time and space they need to give their account, and that they are supported through that process by workers who understand and can normalise reactions that can be quite frightening and disorientating. Having someone available who understands and is able to communicate that they understand the ways this profound shock manifests can provide a much-needed sense of reassurance and safety.

Moreover, a sound grasp of the effects of trauma can also be used by counsellors to advocate for clients—for example, to explain to the police, who often accompany victims in crisis scenarios, why the person may be unable to make a police statement at that point, or decide whether to have

[7] The three typical stress responses are fight, flight and freeze. They are automatic responses (i.e. outside conscious control) promoted by the body's release of stress hormones that occurs after the nervous system detects a threat or danger. In this sequence the amygdala (part of he brains limbic system) activates the body's central stress response system (the hypothalamic pituitary adrenal (HPA) axis which results in the release of neuro-hormones such as adrenaline and cortisol. The adrenaline release results in the heart pumping faster so that more blood gets to the brain and the body, while cortisol suppresses unnecessary functions such as digestive system. While some victims do have a fight or flight reaction the number of victims who know the person who assaults means a freeze reaction is typical reaction. The effect of being assaulted by someone you know often results in a feeling of being destabilized as the person struggles to make sense of what is happening (Haskell & Randall, 2019).

a medical examination, or recall details slowly over time, perhaps not until after they have made their statement. This can play an important part in communicating that the victim is not an 'unreliable witness', deliberately withholding information or being uncooperative; rather; they are presenting in a 'very normal way of coping with and recalling a traumatic experience' (Interview Text No. 27).

For example, the manager cited above (Interview Text No. 23), in continuing to elaborate on the place knowledge about reactions to trauma plays in crisis work, explained how her service had worked with a women who had presented on multiple occasions to undergo a forensic medical examination, each time finding that she was unable to go ahead. The service continued to work with this woman, encouraging her to take the time she needed and advocating for her with the police to ensure pressure was not put on her to make a decision.[8] Eventually, the woman was able to tell the counsellors that each time she presented to have the examination she experienced debilitating flashbacks, not to her recent rape but to the sexual abuse perpetrated by her father during her childhood. The traumatic reactions to that earlier abuse was preventing her from being able to make decisions in relation to her recent rape. Through continuing to work with her at her own pace, the service and counsellors built up sufficient trust that she eventually felt able to tell them about her abuse as a child, and they were able to work with her so that she had sufficient control over her reactions to make a decision. The important point, as this service manager explained, was not what decision the woman made about the forensic medical examination, but that she had the time and space she needed to make that decision, and this was useful in helping to communicate a sense of empathy to the client and in engendering the beginnings of a trusting relationship with the counsellor and with the service.

Conclusion

Feminism and trauma are not, or do not have to be, oppositional forms of knowledge. To the feminist practitioners in this study, key trauma concepts 'made sense', and I have demonstrated how they were able to integrate them into their knowledge/practices. This is not to suggest the integration has been one way, and practitioners represented the uptake of

[8] For the purposes of collecting physical evidence of the assault, the sooner the examination occurs, the stronger the chance of obtaining that evidence.

trauma in the field of sexual assault as both strengthening and altering their feminist practices. However, it does suggest a conceptual compatibility between trauma and feminism. Foucault (1972) uses the term *concomitance* (p. 58) to describe statements, which though they belong to one discourse, they are active within another. These statements may function as a higher authority, acting as either a general principle or premise, an analogous confirmation or a transferable model. For example, relations to philosophy, cosmology and theology defined the discourse of natural history, a fixed classificatory system, and these relations distinguished it from nineteenth-century biology, a discourse based on evolving change over time.

Thus, the integrity of a given discourse may depend on a premise or general principle that is assumed, rather than stated, and akin to an accepted or prior form of knowledge. My conclusion is that there is a concomitant relationship between feminism and trauma, which enables practitioners to integrate trauma into their practice. Practitioners are able to use the neurobiology of trauma as an enabling device because the feminist principle of embodied subjectivity, if not a direct 'fit', at least shares a familial resemblance with the idea that injury to the psyche has a corporeal aspect. Similarly, the representation of sexual assault as an assault on the self and the deployment of trauma as within that representation suggest feminism and trauma share the typical Western ontological concept of an individualised, psychologised self.

In the next chapter (the concluding chapter) I consider the utility of the way trauma has been put to work 'on the ground' for broader feminist thinking about sexual assault. In particular I am interested in beginning to explore the possibility this suggests for making the body, and the embodied harm of sexual violence visible in feminist work on sexual violence.

References

American Psychiatric Association. (1980). *Diagnostic and statistical manual of mental disorders: DSM-III*. Washington, DC: Author.

American Psychiatric Association. (2000). *Diagnostic and statistical manual of mental disorders: DSM-IV-TR* (4th ed., Text rev.). Washington, DC: Author.

American Psychiatric Association. (2013). *Diagnostic and statistical manual of mental disorders: DSM-5* (5th ed.). Washington, DC: Author.

Amir, M. (1968). Victim precipitated forcible rape. *Journal of Criminal Law & Criminology and Police Science, 58*(4), 493–502.

Bourke, J. (2009). *Rape: Sex, violence, history.* Berkeley, CA: Counterpoint.
Bourke, J. (2012). Sexual violence, bodily pain, and trauma: A history. *Theory, Culture & Society, 29*(3), 25–51. https://doi.org/10.1177/0263276412439406
Briere, J. (2002). Treating adult survivors of severe childhood abuse and neglect: Further development of an integrative model. In J. E. B. Myers, L. Berliner, J. Briere, C. T. Hendrix, T. Reid, & C. Jenny (Eds.), *The APSAC handbook on child maltreatment* (2nd ed.). Newbury Park, CA: Sage Publications.
Briere, J., & Scott, C. (2006). *Principles of trauma therapy: A guide to symptoms, evaluations, and treatment.* Thousand Oaks, CA: Sage.
Briere, J., & Scott, C. (2014). *Principles of trauma therapy: A guide to symptoms, evaluation, and treatment* (2nd ed., DSM-5 update ed.). Thousand Oaks, CA: Sage.
Brison, S. (1999). Trauma narratives and the remaking of the self. In M. Bal, J. Crewe, & L. Spitze (Eds.), *Acts of memory* (pp. 39–54). Hanover, NH: University Press of New England.
Brison, S. (2002). *Aftermath: Violence and the remaking of a self.* Princeton, NJ: Princeton University Press.
Bumiller, K. (2008). *In an abusive state: How neoliberalism appropriated the feminist movement against sexual violence.* Durham, NC: Duke University Press.
Burgess, A. W., & Holstrom, L. L. (1974). Rape trauma syndrome. *American Journal of Psychiatry, 13*(9), 981–986.
Burstow, B. (2003). Toward a radical understanding of trauma and trauma work. *Violence Against Women, 9*(11), 1293–1317.
Burstow, B. (2005). A critique of posttraumatic stress disorder and the DSM. *Journal of Humanistic Psychology, 45*(4), 429–445.
Burstow, B. (2015). *Psychiatry and the business of madness: An ethical and epistemological accounting.* New York, NY: Palgrave Macmillan.
Crook, S. (2018). The women's liberation movement, activism and therapy at the grassroots, 1968–1985. *Women's History Review, 27*(7), 1152–1168. https://doi.org/10.1080/09612025.2018.1450611
Cvetkovich, A. (2003). *An archive of feelings: Trauma, sexuality, and lesbian public cultures.* Durham, NC: Duke University Press.
Diamond, D. M., Campbell, A. M., Park, C. R., Halonen, J., & Zolad, P. R. (2007). The temporal dynamics model of emotional memory processing: A synthesis on the neurobiological basis of stress-induced amnesia, flashbulb and traumatic memories, and the Yerkes-Dodson law. *Neural Plasticity*, 60803. https://doi.org/10.1155/2007/60803
Fassin, D., & Rechtman, R. (2009). *The empire of trauma. An inquiry into the condition of victimhood* (R. Gomme, Trans). Princeton, NJ & Oxford: Princeton University Press.
Foucault, M. (1972). *The archaeology of knowledge & the discourse on language* (A. Sheridan, Trans). New York, NY: Pantheon Books.

Gavey, N. (2003). Writing the effects of sexual abuse: Interrogating the possibilities and pitfalls of using clinical psychology expertise for a critical justice agenda. In P. Reavey & S. Warner (Eds.), *New feminist stories of child sexual abuse: Sexual scripts and dangerous dialogues* (pp. 187–209). London: Routledge.

Haaken, J. (1999). Heretical texts: The courage to heal and the incest survivor movement. In S. Lamb (Ed.), *New versions of victims. Feminist struggles with the concept* (pp. 13–41). New York, NY & London: New York University Press.

Haaken, J., & Lamb, S. (2000). The politics of child sexual abuse research. *Society* (May–June), 7–14.

Hart, L. (1998). *Between the body and the flesh. Performing sadomasochism.* New York, NY: Columbia University Press.

Haskell, L., & Randall, M. (2019). *The impact of trauma on adult sexual assault victims*, Department of Justice, Canada. Retrieved from www.justice.gc.ca/eng/rp-pr/jr/trauma/trauma_eng.pdf

Herman, J. L. (1992). *Trauma and recovery: The aftermath of violence - from domestic abuse to political terror.* New York, NY: Basic Books.

Herman, J. L. (2001). *Trauma and recovery. From domestic abuse to political terror.* London: Pandora.

Herman, J. L. (2015). *Trauma and recovery: The aftermath of violence - from domestic abuse to political terror.* New York, NY: Basic Books.

Hunter, S. V. (2010). Evolving narratives about childhood sexual abuse: Challenging the dominance of the victim and survivor paradigm. *The Australian and New Zealand Journal of Family Therapy, 31*, 176–198. https://doi.org/10.1375/anft.31.2.176

van der Kolk, B. (1994). The body keeps the score: Memory & the evolving psychobiology of post traumatic stress. *Harvard Review of Psychiatry, 1*(5), 253–265.

van der Kolk, B. (1997). The psychobiology of posttraumatic stress disorder. *The Journal of Clinical Psychiatry, 58*, 16–24.

van der Kolk, B. (2000). Posttraumatic stress disorder and the nature of trauma. *Dialogues in Clinical Neuroscience, 22*, 1.

van der Kolk, B. (2004). Psychobiology of posttraumatic stress disorder. In J. Panksepp (Ed.), *Textbook of biological psychiatry* (pp. 319–388). New Jersey, NJ: John Wiley & Sons.

van der Kolk, B. (2015). *The body keeps the score: Brain, mind, and body in the healing of trauma.* New York, NY: Penguin Books.

van der Kolk, B., Pelcovitz, D., Roth, S., Mandel, F. S., McFarlane, A., & Herman, J. (1996). Dissociation, affect dysregulation & somatization: The complex nature of adaptation to trauma. *American Journal of Psychiatry, 153*(7), 83–93.

Kozlowska, K., Walker, P., McLean, L., & Carrive, P. (2015). Fear and the defense cascade: Clinical implications and management. *Harvard Review of Psychiatry, 23*(4), 263–287. https://doi.org/10.1097/hrp.0000000000000065

Lamb, S. (1999). Constructing the victim: Popular images and lasting labels. In S. Lamb (Ed.), *New versions of victims: Feminists struggle with the concept* (pp. 108–138). New York, NY & London: New York University Press.

Levett, A. (2003). Problems of cultural imperialism in the study of child sexual abuse. In P. Leavey & S. Warner (Eds.), *New feminist stories of child sexual abuse. Sexual scripts and dangerous dialogues* (pp. 52–76). London: Routledge.

Mardorossian, C. M. (2002). Towards a new feminist theory of rape. *Signs, 27*(3), 743–775.

Marecek, J. (1999). Trauma talk in feminist clinical practice. In S. Lamb (Ed.), *New versions of victims: Feminist struggle with the concept* (pp. 158–182). New York, NY: New York University Press.

O'Dell, L. (2003). The 'harm' story in childhood sexual abuse: Contested understandings, disputed knowledges. In P. Reavey & S. Warner (Eds.), *New feminist stories of child sexual abuse: Sexual scripts and dangerous dialogues* (pp. 131–147). London: Routledge.

Pai, A., Suris, A. M., & North, C. S. (2017). Posttraumatic stress disorder in the DSM-5: Controversy, change, and conceptual considerations. *Behavioral Sciences, 7*(1), 7.

Rose, N. (1996). Critical history and psychology. In C. F. Graumann & K. J. Gergen (Eds.), *Historical dimensions of psychological discourse*. New York, NY: Cambridge University Press.

Rush, F. (1980). *The best kept secret: The sexual abuse of children*. New Jersey, NJ: Prentice Hall.

Schwabe, L. (2017). Memory under stress: From single systems to network changes. *European Journal of Neuroscience, 45*(4), 478–489. https://doi.org/10.1111/ejn.13478

Stark, E. (2007). *Coercive control: How men entrap women in personal life*. New York, NY: Oxford University Press.

Stark, E., Parsons, C., Van Hartevelt, T., Charquero-Ballester, M., McManners, H., Ehlers, A., ... Kringelbach, M. (2015). Post-traumatic stress influences the brain even in the absence of symptoms: A systematic, quantitative meta-analysis of neuroimaging studies. *Neuroscience and Biobehavioural Reviews, 56*, 207–221.

Whittier, N. (2009). *The politics of child sexual abuse. Emotions, social movements and the state*. New York, NY: Oxford University Press.

Wilkin, L., & Hillock, S. (2014). Enhancing MSW students' efficacy in working with trauma, violence, and oppression: An integrated feminist-trauma framework for social work education. *Feminist Teacher, 24*(3), 184–206.

Young, A. (1995). *The harmony of illusions: The invention of post traumatic stress disorder*. Princeton, NJ: Princeton University Press.

CHAPTER 6

Conclusion

Introduction

In this final chapter, I want to explore the possibilities that the ways in which 'the field' has put the neurobiology of trauma to work may offer for feminist theoretical work on sexual violence. In particular, I am interested in exploring the potential that practitioners' engagement with the biological material body—by virtue of the adoption of the neuroscience of trauma—holds for feminist approaches and understandings of sexual violence. Specifically I am interested in the potential this suggests for reintroducing a (non-essentialist) biology of the body into theories of sexual violence. The chapter begins with a brief contextual overview of the place of the body in feminism before sketching possibilities that this uptake of neurobiology in practice suggest for reintroducing the (biological) body into feminist analyses of sexual violence. The chapter concludes with a final reflection of the utility of institutionalised forms of feminism.

The Place of 'the body' in Feminism

Feminism has long kept a wary distance from any engagement with the biology, nature and bodies (Frost, 2014; Warin, 2015). This is understandable given the conflation of the category of woman with biology and nature in western political, legal and social thought and the ways in which this has been used to deny women social, political and economic rights.

S. Egan, *Putting Feminism to Work*,
https://doi.org/10.1007/978-3-030-22109-6_6

Opposition to first wave feminists campaigns for women's right to vote for example was premised on arguments ranging from women's overly emotional temperament, lack of reason and physical strength through to the proposition that women and men naturally inhabited equal but different spheres; the former in the home and the later in the public sphere. The belief that women are somehow '*more biological*, more corporeal, and *more* natural than men' (Grosz, 1994, p. 14) was used even into the twentieth century to deny women access to education, to the professions, from the right to vote, to own property and to manage their own economic affairs. Within this context, it was imperative for feminists to break the deterministic relationship between particular features of women's bodies, their mental capacity and social positions (Lennon, 2019).

The need to break this deterministic relationship, to disentangle women from biological essentialist theories, has perhaps been nowhere more evident than in feminist work against sexual violence. The dominance of the belief in an innate male sexual aggression coupled with the propensity of women's bodies to simultaneously 'provoke' and require such aggression—to achieve sexual satisfaction—made imperative the task of feminists in wresting rape and sexual assault from the realm of the natural and biological. The work of second wave feminists in refiguring of rape as an act of violence rather than as 'just sex', or sex gone wrong was essential to this process (Gavey, 2019). The overarching structure of patriarchy together with the concept of gender provided a framework that shifted the terms of debate from a determinist biologism to one in which the causes of sexual violence are understood to reside in the social and political systems that produce and enable gender inequalities.

This is not to imply that 'the body' per se has been absent from feminist political work. Indeed women's right to control their own bodies has been central to a raft of feminist campaigns from the nineteenth century onwards including the many and ongoing campaigns for reproductive rights (access to birth control, abortion, voluntary motherhood). Likewise, the right of women to bodily integrity, to consent to who touches their bodies and under what circumstances was mobilised in second wave feminist anti-rape women's health campaigns in the 1970s and 1980s and continues as a central motif in much contemporary feminist campaigns and political work (Lennon, 2019).[1] However, as feminist philosopher

[1] For example the slogan 'My Body is Mine' has been used in a number of recent campaigns including in the international feminist organization Mama Cash (2019a) work on

Kathleen Lennon (2019) points out in this type of mobilisation has often been premised on the liberal political philosophy of individual rights, extended to ones right to control one's body. Within this conception, the body exists in a dualistic relationship with the self. It simultaneously exists in relationship to the self, it is an entity over which the self has rights but by virtue of that same relationship is separate from the self.

Moreover, there has been increasing recognition of the extent to which feminist analyses of sexual violence, although developed in response to biologist accounts of rape nevertheless rely on a certain form of biological essentialism. Many feminists writing during this period appear to have accepted the existence of real biological phenomena that differentiated women and men and were used in essentially similar ways across cultures to generate distinctions between males and females and between men and women (Cahill, 2001). Brownmillers (1975), theorisation of sexual violence while based on the concept of patriarchy as a structure and institutional form of male power was never the less example underpinned by the assumption that there are physiological distinctions between male and female bodies that make rape possible. Men have the capacity to rape because they have a penis and women are vulnerable to rape because they have a vagina. In this type of theorisation the biology of bodies remain an unexamined and naturalised substrate on which gender as a social construct, and relations of gender inequality are overlaid.

Conversely, there has been considerable feminist theoretical work on the body over the past twenty years. Associated with the post-structural and linguistic turn that has had increasing purchase across many feminist scholarship from the late 1980s and early 1990s this work has drawn much needed attention to the discursive, representational and disciplinary practices that produce distinctively feminine bodies, disorders and identities.[2] However, as Alaimo and Hekman (2008) highlight, while 'there has been a tremendous outpouring of scholarship on "the body" in the last twenty

women's safety and choice, by ActionAid UK (2020) in their work to stop gendered violence and promote support for survivors and by the Women's Global Network for Reproductive Rights to campaign for the right to safe and legal abortion (WGNRR, 2013). See also Mama Cash (2019b) 'My body is mine: Tracing a feminist slogan'.

[2] Judith Butler's (1990, 1993) work for example helped feminist thinking move past the impasse of the sex/gender binary in which gender as a cultural construct is understood as mapped onto an already sexed body (Wilson, 2015). Rather Butlers work drew attention to the ways in which the performance of gender through discourse produces sexed bodies; that is bodies that are socially and culturally recognised and coded as female or male.

years, nearly all of the work in this area has been confined to the analysis of discourses *about* the body.' (p. 3). Attention to and engagement with the material and biological body has been remained largely absent across many areas of feminist concern (Alaimo & Hekman, 2008; Keane & Rosengarten, 2002; Warin, 2015). Moreover this preoccupation with representation and discourse together with the bracketing or negation of the materiality of bodies such 'makes it nearly impossible for feminism to engage with medicine and science in innovative, productive or affirmative ways—the only path available in the well-worn path of critique' (Alaimo & Hekman, 2008, p. 4). Indeed as Elizabeth Wilson (2002) highlights there has been a certain 'conventionalism surrounding feminist engagement with science which typically 'manifests as the orthodoxy that the biological sciences are politically and conceptually inept, and that the goal of feminist analysis of the sciences is to correct ideological error, rather than to learn from the data that have been produced' (p. 285).

Towards an Engagement with the (Neuro)biology of Bodies

This type of 'conventionalism', I would suggest, encapsulates the position taken in most feminist critique of trauma and sexual violence. The place of feminism in much of this work is positioned as a corrective to the individualised approach of trauma diagnostics by drawing attention to the systemic nature of trauma experienced by oppressed groups and to the structural social inequalities that result in trauma (Burstow, 2003, 2005; Wilkin & Hillock, 2014). Judith Herman's (1992, 2001, 2008, 2015) work in particular is accorded a central role both in extending the trauma framework so that it encapsulates 'private' harms such as domestic violence and drawing attention to the social and political conditions that enable such events to occur (e.g. Griffiths, 2018; Schneider, 2008; Webster & Dunn, 2005).

In this genre of critique, perhaps most overtly encapsulated by the work of radical feminist and anti-psychiatry critic Bonnie Burstow (2015), the concept of psychological trauma is not dismissed; rather, its formalisation as a diagnosis and set of symptoms subject to psychiatric intervention is the focus of a critique. As I laid out in Chapter 5 Burstow (2003, 2005) argues that rather than symptoms of a disorder (PTSD) that the effects be understood as survival strategies and as such are reconceptualised as signs of resilience and strength. Moreover, while critical of formal diagnostics, there is a call by some feminists for understanding a wider range of experiences as traumatic, with a particular focus on the cumulative effects of experiences such as daily encounters with sexism, homophobia and racism, or with poverty. Sometimes referred to as insidious trauma (Root, 1992), this aims to capture the experiences of intimidation and marginalisation that, while they may not be life threatening or overtly violent, over time have a detrimental effect on the individual. Yet there is little acknowledgment of the extent to which this feminist critique or corrective relies on and retains the concept of psychological trauma that is the basis of diagnostic and clinical categories such as PTSD and c-PTSD. The recasting of the symptoms associated with PTSD as survival strategies implicitly relies on ideas, concepts and knowledge (the flashbacks, physiological arousal, numbing, dissociation) that are drawn from medicine, psychiatry and increasingly neuroscience. This disavowal, through the rhetoric of anti-psychiatry, appears not only disingenuous but stymies the possibility of a productive engagement between feminist researchers, theoreticians and practitioners and those from the disciplines in which the concept of trauma originates.

I suggest that consideration of the careful, reflective and active ways in which these practitioners engage with the work of psychiatrists, neuroscientists may provide us with important insights in how to move past the 'conventionalism' (Wilson 2002, p. 285) that has characterised academic feminist engagement with the uptake of sexual assault as trauma. As I have shown that sexual assault workers are highly aware of and conversant with feminist critiques of the medicine and psychiatry. Yet reflecting on their own field of practice this was something that spoken about in the past tense as a position that formed part of their historical narrative rather than a current position. Practitioners were not 'blindly' drawing on the tools of psychiatry or medicine or psychology; rather they had developed a reflective and knowing engagement with these disciplines. There appears both a confidence in the compatibility of a trauma model—whether that be Briere and colleagues (2009, 2010, 2014); Herman (2001, 2015) or van der Kolk (2004, 2015)—with feminist practice and the capacity and skill to draw on each knowledge base as the context and client needs require. As this practitioner highlights below it is about being able to 'pull out' what you need to best work with the particular struggles of a client at that particular moment. There are times when this is best achieved through an explicit evocation of sexual violence as an abuse of gendered power. And there are other moments when knowing how to work with the embodied effects of trauma that need to guide the response.

> So, yeah, I find it's that thing of being able to just pull out when you're with someone, being able to pull out from the bag of tricks what's fitting. So if that person is really struggling with 'I don't understand why I'm sitting at work, nothing's reminding me of this and then I get this flashback', then you pull in more on Briere's stuff. If I'm working with the woman I was describing before, who had a lifetime of sexual assault, she's losing her job from a very high-powered role as a woman. She wanted to talk about the attack, and felt like 'was he trying to bring me down because I was more senior to him'. So then, I'm really drawing on the feminist ideas more strongly, plus some trauma. So it's that thing of being able to pull out whatever [you need] at the time. (Interview Text No. 23)

As I have laid out through the book feminist knowledge of sexual violence—as about gender, power and violence—provides the framework for many enabling practices. It enables practitioners to respond to victims with empathy, to be attuned to the dynamics of power, and to situate individual experiences within a broader social and political context. Yet this framework, as the practitioners pointed out was not always adequate in guiding them through the many practical everyday interactions and difficulties with which victims and survivors present to services. Driven perhaps, by the practical realities that come with having to respond to 'real' individuals presenting with very 'real' material bodily and emotional needs the field of practice shows a productive way to use the knowledge and ideas garnered from trauma to engage with (neuro)biology, material and physical body. They demonstrate a way of recognising the embodied harms and consequences of sexual violence and of engaging with those harms in ways that do not automatically, nor inevitably, render victims and survivors passive, fragile or agentless.

This suggests a way of moving towards a (re)introduction of the body—a non-essentialised biological body—into feminist work on sexual violence. This is important. As I have discussed feminist analyses of sexual violence, based as they are in ideas and concepts derived from second wave feminist analyses of sexual violence do not readily enable an active engagement with the materiality and physicality of the experiences and effects of sexual violence as an embodied experience. Likewise, feminist theoretical work on the discursive and representational body, although of less influence in work against sexual violence appears equally limited. As an example Sharon Marcus (1992) in 'Fighting Bodies, Fighting Words: A Theory and Politics of Rape Prevention' takes feminist sexual violence activism and prevention approaches to task for, even if inadvertently, reproducing rather than ameliorating women's oppression by approaches that represent women as inevitably vulnerable and at risk of sexual violence. As an alternative Marcus (1992) proposes a theory of rape prevention that subverts the traditional 'rape script' by introducing a new language through which we represent women's bodies as active and resistant rather than as wounded inner spaces; and disrupt the construction of the male body as inevitably powerful and untouched by vulnerability. While there is of course merit in developing a different and more expansive language with which to imagine women's bodies, Marcus's theorisation does not extend to or enable an engagement with the materiality and physicality of women's bodies or the embodied effects of sexual violence. Indeed in some respects it relies on the bracketing of the biological body that characterizes feminist theoretical work on sexual violence.

Against this the philosopher Susan Brison (1997, 1999, 2002, 2019) who has drawn on her own experience to think through the theoretical, philosophical, social and cultural issues of sexual violence, highlights not only the profound ways in which the experience fundamentally changed her as a person but the centrality that her body and her changed relationship to her body played in this change.

> I was no longer the same person I had been before the assault, and one of the ways in which I seemed changed was that I had a different relationship with my body. My body was now perceived as an enemy ... and as a site of increased vulnerability. But rejecting the body and returning to the mind was not an option, since the body and mind had become nearly indistinguishable. My mental state (typically, depression) felt physiological, like lead in my veins, whereas my physical state (frequently, one of incapacitation by fear and anxiety) was the incarnation of a cognitive and emotional paralysis resulting from shattered assumptions about my safety in the world. The symptoms of post-traumatic stress disorder gave the lie to a latent dualism that still informs society's most prevalent attitude toward trauma—namely, that victims should "buckup" put the past behind them, and get on with their lives. (1997, pp. 16–17)

Brison's (1997) evocation of the effects of the aftermath of sexual trauma suggest that the effects of sexual violence are embodied in a way that belies any easy distinction between body, mind, and self. Although her body had become 'an enemy' it was no longer possible to take refuge in her mind. Her 'body and mind had become nearly indistinguishable'; physical, emotional and cognitive reactions bound in a recursive loop predicated on the profound changes in understanding of herself and her relationship to the world. In Brison's (1997) account PTSD enables her to make sense of and reconcile herself with the ongoing consequences. Trauma can help in underscoring 'that there is some real harm that has happened to someone, to their bodies, to their beings (Interview Text No. 27).

One of the key criticisms by feminist scholars of the uptake of trauma in feminist work on sexual violence is that this deprives victims of agency. In recent work however Culverhouse (2019) has drawn attention to the extent to which this is underpinned by an assumption that agency resides only in the mind. If a key concern about trauma (PTSD) is that it reduces sexual violence to a medical or mental health problem it is equally underpinned by the long standing suspicion of the way in which mental illness has been equated with biology, in particular the biology of the female body. Using the work of Sharon Lamb (1999) as an exemplar of this particular genre of feminist critique Culverhouse (2019) highlights the way in which PTSD is understood as part of a trend to reverting to biological explanations rather than having to address social responsibilities. PTSD according to Lamb (1999) 'is seen as involuntary and arising from a deep biology of sorts' such that it 'creates the appearance of a victim being victimized by her body, a body that … has somehow turned against her' (p. 112 cited in Culverhouse, 2019, p. 87). Yet as Culverhouse (2019) points out the premise 'that agency is undermined by locating PTSD in the neurobiological and physical aspects of a person reveals an implicit dualism at work, one that risks relegating agency and identity to the mind alone' (p. 87).

Yet it is also possible that recognition of the physicality of trauma via neuroscience—the ways in which it 'lock into the body'—bring with it the possibility of engendering a different understanding of the personhood which does not exist independently of the body nor can be found 'buried beneath layers of skin and bone' (Cahill, 2001, p. 130). Such an understanding opens up possibilities for a different understanding of an agentic self—one which does not rest on an inert biological bodily substrate. Mackenzie and Roberts (2017), in an account of the uptake of neuroscience to inform parenting practices in the field of adoption suggest that the messy context of 'real world' practices' presents a challenge to any easy rejection of this trend as implicitly conservative, biologically reductive or as 'reducible to neoliberal obfuscation or reductionism'(p. 5). Rather they suggest that while this neuroscientific informed—or brain based-approach to parenting can involve elements of determinism it can also involve significant and sometimes seriously helpful shifts in parents' and children's sense

> of agency (moving from personhood based on psychological interiority to one that attempts to figure the brain and brain chemistry and processes as agentic without either relocating the locus of agency to the brain (as causal or determining process) or to biomedicine as the institutional-epistemic embodiment of governing expertise' (Mackenzie & Roberts, 2017, p. 5).

Likewise I am not suggesting that understanding sexual violence through the lens of trauma cannot be used in ways that are unhelpful and problematic. As I laid out in Chapter 5, the concept of complex trauma in particular can be deployed in a manner that reduces problems experienced in adulthood in an overly simplistic linear narrative to sexual victimisation in childhood so that the 'adult survivor 'can appear unable to escape the legacy of such abuse. The concept, however, is capable of enabling effects as demonstrated through its use as a tool to advocate against the poor treatment of victims and to work with survivors to regain a sense of control over the at times debilitating effects that sexual trauma can have on their body/minds, on their relationships and across the full gamut of life. Essentially I have aimed to demonstrate not only that it is not possible—in practice—to reduce the uptake of trauma by sexual assault practitioners to an easy either/or, good/bad, empowering/disempowering, feminist/medicalised. Moreover I suggest that there are productive possibilities for feminist work on sexual violence in considering the way in which the application of trauma in practice brings the body and the embodied consequences of sexual violence to the fore.

Institutionalising Feminism: Final Reflections

The question of feminist engagement with the state (via law reform, working with or within the health, medical and policing systems that respond to sexual violence) is controversial and continues to be the cause of much concern for many feminists (Taylor, 2018). Yet as Whittier (2018) in her analysing the relationships between US feminists and conservatives on the issues of pornography, violence against women and child sexual assault points out, too often debates about working with or targeting the state for change are not based on data about the effects of such efforts. Moreover Sylvia Walby (2011) in work examining the broad policy effects of feminism (for example within projects of the United nations and the European Union) has argued that one of the reasons the strength and vitality of contemporary feminism often goes unnoticed is the extent to which feminism has entered into and become embedded in institutions of civil society and the state, yet continues to be associated with associated with the protest of social movements which implicitly seek public and media attention. While protest, activism and grass roots organising are of course still part of feminism she suggests they tend to occur less frequently such that the less visible work that happens when engaging with the state can lead to the impression that feminism has dissipated or even disappeared.

My interest through this book has been in exploring and making visible what feminism looks like when it moves from this more immediately recognisable grassroots protest and political activism, into the everyday practices and architectural frameworks that make up the field of sexual assault service provision. Approaching feminism as a form of knowledge rather than as an identity (I am feminist or we are a feminist service) or as defined through certain expectations of political activism helped illuminate the almost naturalised position that feminist analyses of sexual violence hold in the field of service provision which formed my object of analysis. Essentially what I have argued for is recognition of the complexity of feminist knowledge, practices and interventions as they play out 'on the ground' in applied contexts. Engaging with sexual violence as a crime, pressing for law reform does not have to mean an absence of or the exclusion of community based preventative work. Working therapeutically with individuals does not have to equate to individualising sexual violence but rather can be ground in a highly politicalised understanding of the relationship between individual experience and structural inequality. Neither does engagement with medical and psychiatric understandings of trauma automatically or unproblematically equate to the 'medicalisation' of sexual violence.

References

ActionAid UK. (2020). Violence against women and girls (VAWG). Retrieved from www.actionaid.org.uk/about-us/what-we-do/violence-against-women-and-girls-vawg

Alaimo, S., & Hekman, S. (2008). Introduction: Emerging models of materiality in feminist theory. In S. Alaimo & S. Hekman (Eds.), *Material feminisms* (pp. 1–19). Bloomington, IN: Indiana University Press.

Briere, J., Hodges, M., & Godbout, N. (2010). Traumatic stress, affect dysregulation, and dysfunctional avoidance: A structural equation model. *Journal of Traumatic Stress, 23*(6), 767–774. https://doi.org/10.1002/jts.20578

Briere, J., & Jordan, C. E. (2009). Childhood maltreatment, intervening variables, and adult psychological difficulties in women: An overview. *Trauma, Violence, & Abuse, 10*(4), 375–388. https://doi.org/10.1177/1524838009339757

Briere, J., & Scott, C. (2014). *Principles of trauma therapy: A guide to symptoms, evaluation, and treatment* (2nd ed., DSM-5 update ed.). Thousand Oaks, CA: Sage.

Brison, S. (1997). Outliving oneself. Trauma, memory and personal identity. In D. Tietjens Meyers, *Feminists rethink the self* (pp. 12–39). Boulder, CO: Westview Press.

Brison, S. (1999). Trauma narratives and the remaking of the self. In M. Bal, J. Crewe, & L. Spitze (Eds.), *Acts of memory* (pp. 39–54). Hanover, NH: University Press of New England.

Brison, S. (2002). *Aftermath: Violence and the remaking of a self.* Princeton, NJ: Princeton University Press.

Brison, S. (2019). Surviving sexual violence: A philosophical perspective. In W. Teays (Ed.), *Analyzing violence against women* (pp. 11–26). Cham, Switzerland: Springer International Publishing.

Brownmiller, S. (1975). *Against our will: Men, women and rape.* London, UK: Secker & Warburg/Simon & Schuster.

Burstow, B. (2003). Toward a radical understanding of trauma and trauma work. *Violence Against Women, 9*(11), 1293–1317.

Burstow, B. (2005). A critique of posttraumatic stress disorder and the DSM. *Journal of Humanistic Psychology, 45*(4), 429–445.

Burstow, B. (2015). *Psychiatry and the business of madness: An ethical and epistemological accounting.* New York, NY: Palgrave Macmillan.

Butler, J. (1990). *Gender trouble: Feminism and the subversion of identity.* New York, NY: Routledge.

Butler, J. (1993). *Bodies that matter: On the discursive limits of "sex".* New York, NY: Routledge.

Cahill, A. (2001). *Rethinking rape.* London, UK: Cornell University Press.

Culverhouse, Z. (2019). From mental illness to moral injury: Psychological and philosophical perspectives on the harm of sexual violence. In W. Teays (Ed.), *Analyzing violence against women* (pp. 81–94). Cham, Switzerland: Springer International Publishing.

Frost, S. (2014). Re-considering the turn to biology in feminist theory. *Feminist Theory, 15*(3), 307–326. https://doi.org/10.1177/1464700114545323

Gavey, N. (2019). *Just sex?: The cultural scaffolding of rape* (2nd ed.). Abingdon, UK and New York, NY: Routledge.

Griffiths, J. (2018). Feminist interventions in trauma studies. In J. R. Kurtz (Ed.), *Trauma and literature Cambridge critical concepts* (pp. 181–195). Cambridge, UK: Cambridge University Press. Retrieved from https://www.cambridge.org/core/books/trauma-and-literature/feminist-interventions-in-trauma-studies/660CF098D8AB47F6E3E5D3B172707910

Grosz, E. (1994). *Volatile bodies. Towards a corporeal feminism.* Sydney, Australia: Allen & Unwin.

Herman, J. L. (1992). *Trauma and recovery: The aftermath of violence - from domestic abuse to political terror.* New York, NY: Basic Books.

Herman, J. L. (2001). *Trauma and recovery. From domestic abuse to political terror.* London, UK: Pandora.

Herman, J. L. (2008). Classics Revisited, Commentary. *Women's Studies Quarterly, 36*(1/2), 282–284.

Herman, J. L. (2015). *Trauma and recovery: The aftermath of violence—From domestic abuse to political terror.* New York, NY: Basic Books.

Keane, H., & Rosengarten, M. (2002). On the biology of sexed subjects. *Australian Feminist Studies, 17*(39), 261–277. https://doi.org/10.1080/0957126022000018070

Lamb, S. (1999). Constructing the victim. Popular images and lasting labels. In S. Lamb (Ed.), *New versions of victims. Feminists struggle with the concept* (pp. 108–138). New York, NY: New York University Press.

Lennon, K. (2019). Feminist perspectives on the body. In E. N. Zalta (Ed.), *The Stanford encyclopedia of philosophy.* Retrieved from https://plato.stanford.edu/archives/fall2019/entries/feminist-body/

Mackenzie, A., & Roberts, C. (2017). Adopting neuroscience: Parenting and affective indeterminacy. *Body and Society. Special Issue on Indeterminacy, 23*(1), 107–127.

Mama Cash. (2019a). My body is mine: Tracing a feminist slogan. Retrieved from www.mamacash.org/en/page/1166

Mama Cash. (2019b). What does # MyBodyisMine mean to you? Retrieved from www.mamacash.org/en/my-body-is-mine

Marcus, S. (1992). Fighting bodies, fighting words: A theory and politics of rape prevention. In J. Butler & J. Scott (Eds.), *Feminists theorize the political* (pp. 385–403). London, UK and New York, NY: Routledge.

Root, M. P. P. (1992). Reconstructing the impact of trauma on personality. In L. S. Brown & M. Ballou (Eds.), *Personality and psychopathology: Feminist reappraisals* (pp. 229–265). New York, NY: Guilford Press.

Schneider, E. M. (2008). Revisiting "Trauma and Recovery". *Women's Studies Quarterly, 36*(1/2), 269–271.

Taylor, C. (2018). Anti-carceral feminism and sexual assault—A defense. *Social Philosophy Today, 34*, 29–49.

van der Kolk, B. (2004). Psychobiology of posttraumatic stress disorder. In J. Panksepp (Ed.), *Textbook of biological psychiatry* (pp. 319–388). New Jersey, NJ: John Wiley & Sons.

van der Kolk, B. (2015). *The body keeps the score: Brain, mind, and body in the healing of trauma.* New York, NY: Penguin Books.

Walby, S. (2011). *The future of feminism.* Cambridge, UK: Polity Press.

Warin, M. (2015). Material feminism, obesity science and the limits of discursive critique. *Body & Society, 21*(4), 48–76.

Webster, D. C., & Dunn, E. C. (2005). Feminist perspectives on trauma. *Women & Therapy, 28*(3–4), 111–142. https://doi.org/10.1300/J015v28n03_06

Whittier, N. (2018). *Frenemies: Feminists, conservatives, and sexual violence.* New York, NY: Oxford University Press.

Wilkin, L., & Hillock, S. (2014). Enhancing MSW students' efficacy in working with trauma, violence, and oppression: An integrated feminist-trauma framework for social work education. *Feminist Teacher, 24*(3), 184–206.

Wilson, E. (2002). Biologically inspired feminism: Response to Helen Keane and Marsha Rosengarten, 'On the biology of sexed subjects'. *Australian Feminist Studies, 17*(39), 283–285. https://doi.org/10.1080/09571260220000018098

Wilson, E. (2015). *Gut feminism.* Durham, NC: Duke University Press Books.

Index

S. Egan, *Putting Feminism to Work*,
https://doi.org/10.1007/978-3-030-22109-6

The manufacturer's authorised representative in the EU is Springer Nature Customer Service Centre GmbH, Europaplatz 3, 69115 Heidelberg, Germany. If you have any concerns regarding our products, please contact ProductSafety@springernature.com

Printed and bound by CPI Group (UK) Ltd, Croydon, CR0 4YY

05/10/2026

02228154-0003